HOME CARE

HOME CARE

A Practical Alternative to Extended Hospitalization

Evelyn M. Baulch

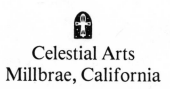

Celestial Arts
Millbrae, California

Celestial Arts
231 Adrian Road
Millbrae, California 94030

First Printing, April 1980

Cover design by Julie Nunes
Drawings in Chapter X are reprinted with permission from *There Is A Rainbow Behind Every Dark Cloud,* © 1978, by The Center for Attitudinal Healing, Tiburon, CA.

Made in the United States of America.

Library of Congress Cataloging in Publication Data

Baulch, Evelyn, 1928–
  Home care.

    1. Home care services. 2. Long-term care of the sick. 3. Home nursing. I. Title [DNLM: 1. Home care services. WY115 B346h]
RA645.3.B38   649.8   79-55665
Hard Cover—ISBN: 0-89087-277-5
Paperback—ISBN: 0-89087-273-2

1 2 3 4 5 6 7 - 86 85 84 83 82 81 80

To Larry: without whom this book would
never have been written

without whom, I would never
have known what love is.

Contents

Acknowledgments

The author wishes to express thanks and to gratefully acknowledge those whose support, advice, experience and expertise made this book possible.

In the beginning when this book was an idea: to Larry, whose illness created the need and whose courage and spirituality provided the foundation for the writing; to my parents, Mr. and Mrs. Armond Miller, for their faithful support and encouragement; to my children, Stephen and Carol Langley, John and Kathy Baulch, and my grandson, Nicholas Langley, for their inspiration; and my close friends, who offered support and good wishes.

To Larry's medical team during his illness: Dr. Irving Katz, Dr. Ronald Lieberman, Dr. Donald Rosenthal, Dr. Lawrence Arnstein; Edna Davis, R.N., Adalyne (Lyn) Allen, R.N., Mary Kirkpatrick, R.P.T., O.T.R., Betty Mobley, R.P.T.; the staff of the Spinal Cord Disability Unit of the Santa Clara Valley Medical Center, and Matthew Desmond, Pharmacist.

To those who permitted me to interview them and to ask questions in the process of preparing the manuscript: Jean Lynn, Aline Fisher, B.A., M.A., C.C.C.; Charlotte Ross, Director of the Suicide Prevention Bureau; Dr. David Levenson, Dr. Richard Carlson, Dr. Gerald Jampolsky, Dr. Ernle Young, Dr. Jim Jett, Dr. Donald Rosenthal; Helaine Dawson, B.A., M.A.; Sharon Winter; Chaplain Walter Johnson, Chaplain Warren Dale and to Ernest Gordon, Dean of the Chapel, Princeton University, for giving us permission to quote from his book, *Through the Valley of the Kwai.* To the patients and families who sought my help and allowed me to share in their experiences.

To Leslie O'Malley, B.A., and Robert Scheid, B.A., M.A., for their research assistance.

To Susan Emigh, R.N., M.A., B.A., for her advice and to Marilyn Stone, R.N., Ph.N., B.S., for reading the entire manuscript and for her expertise and unwavering support.

To my author-friend, Alice Phillips, who helped me edit the manuscript.

To the typists who took over the job of turning my handwritten notes and draft typing into a manuscript: Carol Langley, Helen Koernig, Vickie Auguston, Sue Burns, Monica Bosch and Susan Kashack.

To my agent, Deborah Johansen, who read the original writing and had confidence in me and in the publication of my work.

To my attorney, Brian Gill, for his friendship and legal advice.

To my editor, Joycelyn Moulton, who lovingly and expertly turned a typed manuscript into a book and to Celestial Arts Publishing Company for turning my dream into a reality.

And finally, I thank Almighty God, who produced and directed my efforts.

Preface

It was a lovely May morning in 1976 and I sat propped up on pillows on the waterbed in our home. Beside me lay my husband, Larry, bedridden and partially paralyzed. We were indulging in our long-time morning ritual, reading and discussing articles in the morning paper. Suddenly, there was an interruption.

Larry had always said that an interruption was an opportunity, and he was right. Our casual enjoyment of the news was interrupted when we read and became engrossed in an article advocating home care for seriously ill patients and stressing the importance of the family as a positive influence. The opportunity (although we didn't know it then) was this book, which outlines what we learned about that subject in the more than four years we shared Larry's illness.

The first draft of the book, yet unborn, was a simple list of helpful suggestions that Larry and I drew up to give to friends who asked for some guidance in their similar experiences. It went through a number of expansions and was given to people referred to us by Larry's fellow ministers and to the flood of strangers who called us after a local newspaper published an article on our home care adventure.

For us, home care was not an alternative. It was normal. We both hated the separation of Larry's intermittent hospitalization. We missed the intimacy of our morning newspaper discussion, for one thing. We were also convinced that the positive influence of the home with family and friends dropping by was enormous. And, in the face of rising hospital costs, it was much less expensive.

I am not a medical professional. Patients and their families seldom are. I am a secretary, but I had been able to learn the mechanics of home care; Larry, as a minister, was able to deal with many of the psychological and emotional problems involved. We were not special, and we felt that if we could do it—and we did—anyone could handle it.

Much has been written by professionals that has great merit and I strongly urge that you read and take advice from those with good medical and nursing knowledge, sound psychological advice and powerful spiritual insights. The bibliography at the end of this book has been compiled as a guide to your further reading.

This book is about people. All of us are connected by our mutual human vulnerability. We will all be sick at some time. And certainly we will all die. This book describes some of our common experiences, experiences that we now have or will have in the future. This is my story of home care, of Larry and my efforts to care for him. I

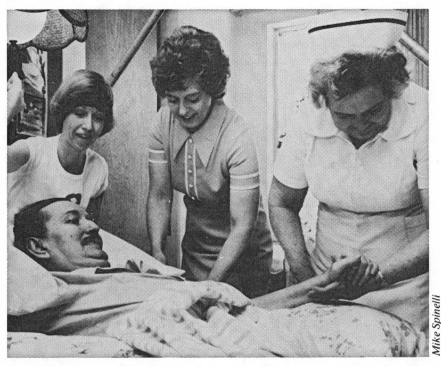

Mike Spinelli

The author, Evelyn M. Baulch, is pictured working as part of the home care team. In foreground, Larry Baulch, the patient and leader of the team; left to right, Mary Kirkpatrick, physical therapist, Evelyn Baulch and Lyn Allen, R.N.

have interviewed patients and their families, doctors, nurses, health care professionals, and members of groups in the community who can offer you assistance. Your experience will be different in some ways because you are another human being and you will have your own unique needs. But the process of providing home care for someone who is ill or injured has basic rules and functions applicable to everyone.

This book describes the practicalities of home care, the choices that families have when a long-term illness is being faced, the physical and emotional drain home care may entail, and the joys and satisfaction it can bring. It was written to be used as a resource for families facing the agony of long-term illness or injuries. It was designed to start with the first shock of diagnosis and carries through in a somewhat chronological order. Chapter headings will serve as a guide and index for readers searching for help in particular areas. It will be most helpful when used as a reference book.

Larry's long bout with cancer and, finally, partial paralysis forced us to live on a different level. We were always close when he was well, but his illness brought us into a deeper relationship, one that we could not have attained had he remained healthy. Our perspectives changed and we were carried into a higher form of humanity: that of one person caring for another. The limitations of his illness compelled us to find new ways of relating to each other and to all those whose lives we touched.

I look back on the experience home care gave us with gratitude and joy and as a time when a devastating interruption became a remarkable opportunity. It is my hope that if you sometime face such an interruption in your life, something in this book will help you.

I believe in home care and I am committed to the process of healing—in the holistic sense—whether it be of the body, mind or spirit.

Evelyn M. Baulch

HOME CARE

Chapter I

Where to Begin

Life is what happens to you while you are planning something else.

. . .A young man, celebrating his graduation from high school dives into the river, strikes bottom and sustains an injury that renders him a paraplegic.

. . .A middle-aged woman discovers a lump in her breast as she showers in preparation for her daughter's wedding.

. . .A retired businessman on his first vacation in years slumps over the table of a fashionable restaurant. His heart attack changes his retirement plans from travel to immobility.

All of these people were planning something else. Certainly, they were not arranging to become statistics in the ever-increasing numbers of people who require long-term, perhaps life-term, care.

To each of them the knowledge came suddenly, almost without warning. In virtually all cases, it came without the victim being prepared for the calamity.

The path to medical treatment begins abruptly. Health crises are not planned, seldom expected. If they are given any thought at all it is only that such things happen to other people. You are never prepared to have it happen to you or someone you love.

In the majority of cases, the message is delivered to the patient or his family in a hospital setting. Either he has been sent there by a doctor ordering tests, or brought to the emergency room after an accident or medical emergency.

Let us assume that the original trauma has been dealt with and you are now facd with long-term medical treatment, care and/or therapy.

1

START WITH A DOCTOR

The medical world is controlled by doctors. You cannot be admitted or officially released from a hospital except by a physician's order. While you are there, the doctor orders and supervises all treatment, including diagnostic tests. You cannot get the medication you need after release from the hospital without a doctor's prescription. But most importantly, you *need* the best medical advice you can get from a doctor.

Your problems will be lightened considerably if you have a personal physician, one you know well and trust, one who knows you. Since this is something that cannot be achieved on the spot, I urge anyone who is not in immediate crisis and who does not have a personal or family physician to take care of that situation immediately. It is one of the few things you can do to prepare for an unexpected illness or injury.

Everyone should have a family doctor trained in either general practice or internal medicine. You need one doctor to whom you can refer all your medical problems. He in turn will advise you if you need to see a specialist.

If you do not have a doctor, you will need to shop for one. Ask a friend whose opinion you value highly for a recommendation. You can also call your local medical society, which is listed in the telephone directory. Outline your requirements. They will give you the name of several doctors appropriate for your needs in your area. Further information concerning a physician's age, education, residency, length and location of practice, and specialties is usually available in the Directory of Physicians published by the American Medical Association or the Directory of Medical Specialists published by the American Board of Medical Specialties (of which Family Practice is now included as a medical specialty). These volumes are generally available in major libraries through the reference desk or in the libraries of medical societies.

The most important requirement for a doctor is good, open communication. You must feel confident that the doctor understands your problems and will honestly advise you concerning your care.

Communication is a two-way exchange. If you want good advice from the doctor, you must be very explicit in what you convey to him. He can only evaluate and answer questions in terms of what you tell him. Your doctor does not operate with a crystal ball. He cannot understand thoughts, doubts, or information that you do not communicate.

If you have a feeling the doctor is not understanding what you have said, you are probably right. Rephrase and repeat, but do not let the interview end unless you are satisfied. If you do not feel comfortable with the doctor and you do not have total trust in him, I would suggest you find another.

It is important to know that the doctor works for you. You hire him to do a job for you. He provides a service for which you are charged. If you do not receive the service you request you simply let the doctor know that you have decided to take your case to another physician. Then request that copies of all your records be transferred to the new doctor you have selected.

ASK QUESTIONS

The interview with the doctor should be held with the patient and the family together, if possible. It is important from the very beginning to have total honesty in all relationships. The most frequent complaint I hear from patients is that they are afraid information is being withheld from them, either by the doctor or the family. Sometimes their fears are more destructive than the truth would be. Patients develop a strong intuitive sense. They often discern their true condition from the attitudes of those around them.

If the patient is in a coma, or if for some other medical reason cannot meet with the doctor, the closest family member or members will need to ask questions. They should share the information with the patient as soon as it is appropriate to do so.

Not only is it wise to ask questions, you now have a legal right to question. Under recent legislation called Informed Consent, doctors must advise patients—or the family if a patient is unconscious—of the nature of the illness or injury, options for treatment and risks involved. This consent becomes a part of the patient's medical records. The doctor may advise or recommend but the decision concerning treatment belongs totally to the patient.

The Questions

Make a list of your questions before you meet with the doctor. It is difficult to remember everything so be prepared to jot down his answers to your questions, too.

If you do not know what to ask, here are some examples.
1. What is the disease or injury for which the patient is being treated? Get specifics on this. Don't accept generalities. If it is

cancer, what kind of tumor is it and where is it located? What has been the most successful treatment? What are the side effects of the suggested treatment? In the case of stroke or injury, what areas are affected? Is damage permanent or temporary?

2. Get exact names of medications, surgical procedures, infections, treatment. It is not enough to know that the patient is "being treated for an infection." Find out what kind of infection, where it is located, how it is being treated, and what medication is being given.
3. What treatment is the patient receiving? Get names of medications, dosage, and possible side effects.
4. Is full recovery possible? Can the doctor give you an indication of when full recovery might be expected?
5. Will there be any permanent impairment?
6. What follow-up care is needed? Is any kind of therapy indicated?
7. What does the doctor advise?
8. Date of release, provided no complications occur?

If your physician is a general practitioner or an internist he may refer the patient to other specialists. If the patient has been injured in an accident he may need the services of an orthopedic surgeon or a plastic surgeon. A heart attack patient would most likely be referred to a cardiac specialist. Cancer patients may need the services of a surgeon, radiologist or chemotherapist.

Ask questions. You may want a second opinion. Good doctors understand this and do not feel threatened by consultations. Oftentimes doctors themselves suggest that you get a second opinion if there are unusual symptoms, treatment or diagnosis.

When Larry had his original testing and received a diagnosis of cancer in the right kidney from a urologist, we asked for a second opinion from another urologist. The first doctor encouraged us to seek a second opinion and arranged to have all tests, X rays, and lab results made available to the doctor we selected. The second doctor concurred with the original diagnosis and recommended that Larry have surgery immediately. The second opinion did not change the outcome in our case, but we felt more confident about having surgery.

You should be prepared in the event you receive conflicting opinions. If this happens, you may need to get a third doctor to review the case.

In order to make decisions, you need the best, most competent professional advice you can get. But whether you have the advice of one doctor, two, three, or more—the final decision is always yours.

Chapter II

What Choices Do You Have?

A hospital stay is a dramatic interruption in a person's life. Most people stay in the hospital for only a few days and return home to a normal, healthy life. But for some, who are seriously ill or injured, the stay is longer and they still need special care after their hospital confinement.

There comes a time when a decision must be made as to where the patient will go when released from the hospital. In order to make choices you need to know what kinds of care are available.

TYPES OF CARE

Acute Care Facilities
Certain hospitals and university teaching centers maintain life support care which includes emergency treatment, surgery, and crisis care by doctors and nurses on duty twenty-four hours a day. X ray and laboratory work are done on the premises. Out-patient treatment may also be provided.

Skilled Nursing Facilities
These facilities, which may be called extended care or convalescent homes in some areas, are operated with twenty-four hours professional nursing staff on duty. Doctors are called as needed. This type of facility provides care for a wide range of patients, usually those who need long-term care such as the elderly, patients who are bedridden, and patients with disabilities. They provide special dietary supervision and physical, occupational, speech and recreational therapy.

5

Intermediate Care Facilities
Some facilities are licensed for a less intense level of care than the skilled nursing facilities. Patients may or may not be ambulatory but must be able to do many things for themselves and require minimal skilled care.

Residential Care Facilities
These facilities are generally operated without professional staff on the premises. Doctors and public health nurses are called as needed. Patients who live in these homes usually must be ambulatory, able to care for their own bodily functions, and be mentally alert. In most states homes with more than one person are required to be licensed.

Rehabilitation Centers
Such facilities are staffed by professionals who provide multiple therapies and/or counseling. Some larger centers are connected to acute care facilities where reconstructive and/or rehabilitative surgery are also performed.

Home Care
The patient's care is supervised by his or her doctor with nursing care provided by family or professionals as needed. Home physical therapy can be arranged.

If the patient is a veteran, check with the Veterans Administration for benefits and advice about special services and facilities.

If you already receive public assistance benefits, check with the local Social Security or County Welfare Agency. You may be entitled to disability or other benefits.

SEE A DISCHARGE PLANNER

If your hospital staff includes a discharge planner, by all means avail yourself of this new and helpful service. Their main concern is the patient and her specific needs.

The discharge planner can provided objective counseling on the type of care that will be needed and the financial arrangements that are available. They can review the patient's private insurance coverage, discuss possible state aid and Medicare benefits, disability benefits through private insurance, Workmen's Compensation, state and federal agencies. If a patient expects to pay for her own care, she will be able to discuss costs of treatments with the planner.

If the hospital has no discharge planning service, contact the local Family Service Agency (also known as the Family Service Association of America). It is a national, nonprofit organization providing many kinds of services with sliding scale fees and referral services to other agencies. Look for it under "F" for Family Service in the white pages of your telephone directory. Home-care agencies are available in some communities to assist patients and families who feel home to be the most desirable environment for convalescence.

Other social service agencies you might contact are the Catholic Social Service, Lutheran Social Service, Jewish Family and Children's Agency, and Crippled Children's Service, which are usually listed in a telephone directory of metropolitan areas.

Another helpful source of information is the reference desk of local libraries. Oftentimes they are equipped with a computerized referral service that provides information on many subjects. Questions can be programmed into the computer and information is at your fingertips.

At the very least, they will provide a directory of the national offices addresses of organizations to which you can write for further information concerning facilities and services in your area. It is not unusual in rural areas for health care services and therapies to be available through visits from staff of the agency in the nearest large city, but the contact usually must be initiated by the patient, her family or physician.

The library is also a good source of lists of residential and skilled care facilities. Armed with lists, you will want to call first to determine availability of space, then visit them to compare services, atmosphere, staff, size and whether they meet your particular needs.

Use Community Agencies As Resource

Depending on what kind of illness or injury your patient has suffered, some agencies to call for assistance are:
   Heart Association
   Kidney Foundation
   Multiple Sclerosis Society
   American Cancer Society
   Easter Seal Society
   March of Dimes

The American Heart Association is a national organization with local chapters. The organization provides money for research in heart disease and offers community programs such as diet counseling, hypertension screening and cardiopulmonary resuscitation training. Films, brochures and speakers are usually available to the public.

Some chapters have full time dieticians on the staff who counsel patients about diet, and hold diet modification workshops to educate the general public in diet control for the prevention of hypertension and to reduce the risk of heart disease. Hypertension screening is another community service: blood pressure is checked at county fairs and shopping centers in an effort to alert potential victims to the dangers of high blood pressure. A person must be aware he has high blood pressure (one of the major causes of strokes) before he will seek help from a doctor.

Frequently, volunteers who have had heart disease work with patients who are diagnosed as having heart disease. In some areas there are Mended Heart Groups which meet monthly. The volunteers (who are post heart surgery people) work with others who are facing heart surgery. They also cosponsor such activities as A Stroke Club, Parents for Heart Club (made up of parents who have children with heart disease), and conduct classes in cardiopulmonary resuscitation (their aim is to train ten percent of the total population to support life until medical help can be obtained.)

The Easter Seal Society is a national organization with local chapters which provide programs and services for handicapped children and adults. Some chapters have rehabilitation centers and workshops, social service departments for counseling, pools for therapy treatment, and provide both speech and occupational therapy. The workshops, which employ handicapped persons, work with industry on a subcontract basis. Agencies loan equipment (wheelchairs, walkers, etc.) to handicapped people as one of their services. The National Easter Seal organization also sponsors research and promotes legislation to help the handicapped.

The National Multiple Sclerosis Society has local chapters that provide money for research (no cause or cure for MS is known), provide public education materials and films (professionals and nonprofessionals help), and have programs and assistance for the patient and family. Counseling is available, there is an equipment loan program, some attendant care is provided in case of emergency, transportation is available, and an MS auxiliary plans occasional activities. They mail a quarterly newsletter and have films available for public use.

The American Cancer Society is a national organization with local chapters. It provides a program of public information on early detection of cancer including the seven danger signals and breast examinations, and encourages peolpe to quit smoking: "Being A Quitter" stop smoking club. In some areas crisis counseling on a short-term basis is provided by a medical social worker. Sickroom equipment is usually loaned free of charge and discounts arranged if they do not have the equipment on hand and the patient needs to buy items, but this must be arranged in advance of purchase. Some chapters provide free bandages and surgical dressings and also transportation through volunteers called Free Wheelers for patients who require this kind of service.

Rehabilitation services include the Reach For Recovery program for mastectomy patients. Trained volunteers who have had breast surgery visit new patients before and after surgery to offer emotional support and practical information. Ostomy patients visit new ostomy patients and Laryngectomee Club members also visit new patients. Kits which include information and helpful materials are provided for the patient and delivered by the volunteer. Speech therapy is provided at no charge by a qualified speech therapist for laryngectomy patients. The American Cancer Society also has an active program for cancer research.

March of Dimes is a national foundation dedicated to preventing birth defects and alleviating their destructive consequences. It supports a broad range of programs in research, perinatal and genetic medicine, professional and public health education and community services. Birth defects include mental retardation, blindness, deafness, missing limbs, defective blood cells, and body chemistry disorders.

The National Kidney Foundation has volunteer leadership seeking an answer to prevention, treatment, management and cure of kidney disease. They encourage and promote research, cooperate with public and private agencies in services for persons suffering from the disease, provide community education about the many aspects of kidney disease (including symposiums and conferences,) and formulate local and federal legislation to assist patients in obtaining services, and improving research programs.

The Gift Of Life program was formed to try to locate donors for kidney transplants. Twenty-eight states now have legislation allowing people to indicate on their drivers' licenses that they wish to be donors. There is often a difficulty in tissue match and appropriate donors. This program seeks to aid those persons waiting for transplants.

It's worth a phone call; these agencies are a good source of information and assistance. Services may vary from area to area as local chapters provide services to meet the needs of their communities. But no matter where you live, some help is available in your own city or nearby.

The hospital discharge planner's office generally has a supply of printed information on specific problems (cancer, strokes, etc.), schedules of out-patient classes for heart and diabetic patients, and information on facilities available for residential or extended post-hospital care. A planner will generally suggest other agencies for further assistance.

No one need do without care because of lack of money; funding is available for some kind of care for everyone.

THE CASE FOR HOME CARE

In this day of a society that has become institutionally oriented, home care is generally considered as an option or an alternative to hospital or institutional care.

I do not agree. I believe that home care is the normal environment for the patient and that all other facilities are the alternatives to being at home.

Home care provides the most normal atmosphere, a comfortable and familiar environment for the patient. Serious illness and injuries are in themselves depressing; removal from the warmth and security of the home can only make the depression deeper.

The services a patient would receive in the hospital are not precluded by home care. Under supervision of the doctor, a nurse may visit the home to administer drugs, check blood pressure and train the family in care procedures. Medical equipment and supplies are readily available and the patient may receive therapy at home.

Home care has the unqualified support of the American Cancer Society. As a result of a study initiated in 1973, the Society has published a booklet that describes the advantages, from a psychological and rehabilitative standpoint, of home care calling it "of significant benefit to families and patients needing only intermittent care."

Sylvia Porter, nationally syndicated economist, advocating the various home care insurance programs now available, had this to say in a February, 1978 column, "Home health care programs are taking hold from coast to coast as one of the 'newest' solutions to runaway hospital costs (although, in actuality, home care is the oldest form of care there is.) Today, 55 of the nation's 70 Blue Cross plans offer home care benefits to more than 33 million of their subscribers, against only 25 million subscribers in 32 plans six years ago."

Later in another column devoted to studies made by Blue Cross and Blue Shield Company, she continued, "In fact, documented studies show that Blue Cross home health care plans save 10.2 to 18.5 hospital days per case, with dollar savings per case running from $330 to over $900."

HOW WE GOT AWAY FROM HOME CARE

There was a time when people were totally responsible for their own care. Treatment, such as it was, was given at home by the family or other members of the community. The first hospitals grew out of the centers established by religious orders for sick, weary travelers in the early Christian era. For centuries they served only those who were too sick or too poor to be cared for at home. Even then, doctors did not work in these institutions but treated patients at home.

Although the concept of hospitals was more than a thousand years old, European hospitals in the early seventeen hundreds were still maintained for the poor. The well-to-do were cared for at home.

Two discoveries, the principles of antisepsis and the use of ether as an anesthetic during surgery, in the first half of the nineteenth century led to the trend of caring for patients in hospitals instead of at home. The use of X-ray equipment, the creation of nursing schools and the idea of private rooms for patients followed quickly and the charity hospital image began to diminish.

The trend continued, strengthened by hospitalization insurance, first offered in 1929, and was given another boost when the lag in hospital building, created by the Depression, was turned around by federal funds during World War II. The rapid growth of hospitals since then has been toward bigger and therefore more impersonal institutions. Coupled with these vast medical centers is the proliferation of specialization, further reducing patient-physician relationships.

Thus has grown the use and importance of hospitals to the point that what once was an option to home care has become its complete replacement.

Today we can have the best of both worlds, if we will use them—the technology of modern medicine as practiced in a hospital environment, and the intimacy and warmth of home care where the patient can remain a part of the family unit.

Chapter III

Making the Decision
on Post Hospital Care

The earlier you start making plans for care after hospitalization the more time you will have to implement the choice you make. Under normal conditions you will have a few days to make this decision and you already have some of the information on which your choice will be made.

You will have:
1. selected a doctor,
2. a clear understanding of the diagnosis and prognosis.
3. asked the doctor's advice about post hospital care and continued treatment.
4. talked with a discharge planner or social worker and know your financial health care benefits.
5. become aware of the types of care available.

The two final and most important factors to consider are:

what the patient wants, and

what the family wants and can realistically provide.

The patient's needs and desires should be considered first, because her recovery and quality of life during her illness depend a great deal on mental attitude. If her desires cannot be fully met, it is still best if she can participate in the discussion and make a decision for an alternative compromise.

The patient should be asked straight out what she wants to do. This is a time when a solid relationship is needed. If she says, "You might as well put me in a convalescent home because I'll never get any better," you must understand that she probably isn't expressing

13

honest feelings. It is a reply meant to give you an "out." No one wants to become a burden on their family.

Larry, who I knew wanted to be home, would make a statement like this occasionally. I realized it was an effort on his part to give me the chance to give up his care if I wanted. I had to be certain that I was being honest with my own feelings when I said, "I want you home, no matter how hard it is." I knew I had to mean it. He would have known if I had been dishonest with him.

The second consideration is an assessment of the total family's needs and desires. Families must evaluate their strengths and weaknesses in terms of time available for care, physical home facilities, financial assets and health care benefits, emotional attitude about illness, and spiritual strengths. How much care can the family reasonably provide?

If a wife doesn't want to do home care, for instance, she should determine whether her reluctance is based on her own doubts of her ability to do a good job—which could be overcome by support and training—or whether she honestly does not want to take the responsibility. If the latter is the case, she could not do home care effectively. Her reluctance would have a negative effect on the patient. A better choice might be to choose either a residential or skilled care facility. She could then support that care.

Job requirements might limit the amount of care that could be provided. An example was the case of Anna, a middle-age stroke victim with some impairment of function who could have been cared for at home. She was, in fact, quite eager to go home. Her husband, however, had a job that required considerable travel so he was unable to provide care himself. They chose a skilled care facility on a temporary basis while extensive therapy was given and later arranged for professional nursing care at home.

Sometimes finances limit the choices for patients, but they should still participate in the decision rather than being told what they must do.

The facilities must also be considered. We made many changes to accommodate Larry's care. In fact, after he became paralyzed we sold our house because we could not get his wheelchair up and down the steep driveway. We rented a duplex apartment, all on one level, where Larry had access to the entire house and could go out to the car via a ramp or into the patio unassisted.

You may find that your living quarters are not satisfactory. Questions about how to make changes in your present living accommodations are discussed more fully in the next chapter. For now, it is only important to be aware of the possible need for changes and begin thinking about how they might be accomplished in your situation.

Be sure your care goals are realistic.

Some choices are easier to make than others. The patient may have only a short-term impairment: for example, broken bones may be an inconvenience but doctors can predict the recuperation period. Families that have had previous experience with treatment and care will be better prepared to analyze and solve the problem.

Those faced with a more difficult prognosis or without previous experience will need to seek the advice of medical professionals to assure that choices they have made about the type of care they want are realistic. For instance, a doctor might advise that a patient go to a rehabilitation facility or skilled care facility for a short period of time before going home.

Patients are generally eager to go home. They may insist on being released before their care has been planned, or they may want to go home when home care is not realistically one of the options, due to financial considerations, family limitations or the patient's condition. In these cases, you will need the strong support of the doctor (or other health care professional) to objectively discuss the situation and to help the patient clarify more reasonable goals.

Elderly patients may want to return home, but they may not have a family to provide home care and they may not have health care insurance benefits to cover the cost of home nursing.

It is important to remember that the choice you make now is not irrevocable.

If your plan doesn't work, change it. You may try one kind of care facility and find it unsatisfactory. You may need to make other choices as the patient's condition, finances or family situation changes. If you are aware of your alternatives in types of care and care facilities, you can move with the changes.

I have had experience with all five types of care and have made decisions to move a family member from one kind to another. In Larry's case, we did home care the majority of the time, but when he needed tests, laboratory work, X rays and surgery we went to an acute care hospital where he was treated for a few days or weeks and then came home again. After one spinal surgery he was sent to a spinal cord disability unit for rehabilitative therapy before returning home.

My grandmother was home until she was eighty-three years old. Medical problems necessitated a move to a residential care facility. About two years later she was admitted to an acute care facility for emergency surgery for a broken hip. Her change in condition required admission to a skilled care facility upon release. She is now ninety years old and within the seven-year period from the time home care was no longer an option she has been moved to alternative facilities which could provide the best care possible considering her condition at a particular time.

Don't let little decisions keep you from making the big decision.

Make the decision on which type of care is more appropriate first; then you can make the other decisions needed to implement the kind of care you have chosen.

Let's review those basic choices again:

If the patient is:

> *In hospital now:*
> Choices: go to skilled care facility
> go to residential care facility
> go to rehabilitation facility
> go home

> *In skilled care facility now:*
> Choices: go to acute care facility
> go to residential care facility
> go to rehabilitation facility
> go home

> *In a residential care facility now:*
> Choices: go to acute care facility
> go to skilled care facility
> go to rehabilitation facility
> go home

At home now:

Choices: go to acute care facility
               go to skilled care facility
               go to residential care facility
               go to rehabilitation facility

In a rehabilitation facility now:

Choices: go to skilled care facility
               go to residential care facility
               go to acute care facility
               go home

You may want to return to a discharge planner for assistance in implementing your decision, for help in completing insurance forms and advice on how to locate local care facilities.

If you have decided to do home care: you can begin by making preparations prior to the patient's release.

If you have decided to use a residential care facility, or skilled facility: you will need to begin looking for an appropriate place.

Chapter IV

What You Need to Do
before Hospital Release

Once your doctor has given you a date for hospital discharge, you should have from five to seven days in which to prepare for the move. If you have less than that and feel you will not be able to make adequate arrangements you may ask your doctor to add a few days to the hospital stay.

INSTITUTIONAL CARE

If you have elected institutional care your major task is to locate the proper facility of a type your doctor has already advised you is best suited to care for the patient.

You will also need to arrange transportation to that facility and take home everything the patient is not using before release date.

ARRANGE TRANSPORTATION

Unless the patient is able to be moved in a car you will need to arrange for an ambulance. This should be done no later than the day before release, earlier if possible. Some services have van-type vehicles that can load a patient in a wheelchair.

Most hospitals observe an 11:00 A.M. release time. Patients not moved until afternoon or evening will be charged for an extra day. Check with the cashier ahead of time to verify the time and also for other discharge requirements. In any case you will need to visit the cashier to arrange payment.

When Larry was hospitalized I usually arranged for an ambulance at 9:30 A.M., which gave him time to have an unhurried breakfast and gave us a margin of time before the 11:00 A.M. checkout time.

TAKE EVERYTHING HOME

Even a short stay in the hospital results in an accumulation of flowers and plants, gifts, books and magazines, get-well cards and notes. They may take up more space and be trickier to move than the patient himself.

Since Larry had surgery a number of times I've had lots of occasions to sit in hospital lobbies and I often saw families struggling with the last-minute details of moving a patient and of making a half-dozen trips up and down the elevator carrying everything from flowers to fruit while the patient waited uneasily in a wheelchair.

It is usually easier to take a few things home each day, leaving only things that will be needed for the last night's stay. Those few items can be dropped in a bag in a moment and whisked off to the car along with the patient. Easier on you; less confusion to tire the patient.

GOING HOME

For those who have made the home-care decision there is more preparation. To begin with, keep in mind that basically you will need to continue the same care that is being given by the hospital staff. Start now to learn all you can about that care. As much as possible become a part of his care team. Note how beds are made, how a pull sheet makes moving the patient easier, both for him and for the nurse, how he is bathed. Don't be afraid to ask questions, learn about his diet, medication and as many of the small but important details of the care he needs as you can.

How smoothly things run after a patient arrives home will depend on how well you prepare yourself beforehand. Arranged in their priority are some things you will need to do to assure a smooth transition from hospital to home.

1. Arrange for follow-up care from a doctor. Get complete written instructions about treatment and medications.

2. Ask if medications will be provided by the hospital to take home or if you will need to have prescriptions filled. Determine where you will purchase medicine.

3. Arrange for nursing care.

4. Arrange for physical therapy/occupational or speech therapy, if needed.
5. Make preparations of the home to facilitate continuing care.

6. Purchase supplies. Rent, buy or borrow equipment needed.

7. Devise your own patient chart for recording care and treatment.

8. Take home everything the patient is not using prior to release.

9. Arrange for patient's transportation.

1. Arrange for Follow-up Care from a Doctor

By this time you should have a doctor or doctors supervising care. You need to arrange for follow-up care either at home or in another facility if the patient cannot go to a doctor's office for checkups. Some doctors work only from their office. If the doctor you are using does not make house calls, you will need to find a doctor who does.

You may need more than one doctor. For example, surgery will require follow-up care by the surgeon or perhaps you will need the supervision of a physical therapy specialist. You may need to consult other doctors at various times. It is important, however, that one doctor have primary responsibility, with other doctors serving as consultants.

After you have selected the one doctor to supervise care, you should establish a definite schedule for visits and phone calls. More frequent visits may be necessary during the first weeks after hospital confinement, followed by semimonthly or monthly examinations thereafter.

Phone calls should be made to the doctor when any circumstance warrants. It is better to make a phone call immediately to the doctor if something seems wrong than to delay and risk complications. Always give the doctor complete factual information or ask precise questions so he will be better able to evaluate the situation.

Ask the doctor to give you written instructions for post hospital care, treatment and medications. Keep these instructions with your home-care chart (see item #7, "Chart"). You will need to have the doctor's orders available at all times. As care progresses, the instructions and medications may change. Be sure to get all changes in writing.

Always keep the original sheets of instructions. *Do not throw anything away.* You may need to refer to them at some later time.

The first day at home is a busy one so have the doctor's prescriptions filled in advance of release so that the medication is on hand when the patient arrives home.

2. Know Your Pharmacist

While hospital pharmacies are more convenient, their charges are usually higher than at other pharmacies. Take a few minutes to do some comparative shopping. Pharmacies are required by law to provide a list of prices for prescription drugs. If not displayed, ask the pharmacist for prices. You may want to save time by calling several pharmacies.

You will probably not be able to read the prescription itself, but you can get the names of the medications from the doctor's written instructions. Pharmacists will be able to give you the price of each medication. Prescriptions for long-term use are usually less expensive if you buy in quantity.

Another way to save money is to ask your doctor to prescribe drugs by their generic rather than brand name, as they are considerably cheaper. Not all drugs, however, have a generic equivalent.

If you plan to do consumer shopping by telephone, please be considerate of the pharmacist's time. Avoid calling after 4:00 P.M. on weekdays and on weekends when most pharmacists are the busiest.

Discount drug stores usually offer the lowest prices for prescriptions. If saving money is your most important consideration, you may decide to buy from them. If you need home delivery of medications, you will pay a slightly higher price for this service. Geographical location is another consideration. You may prefer to buy from a drug store conveniently located near your home, which has easy access and parking space available, as opposed to a discount store located across town.

I decided to use a pharmacy conveniently located within two blocks of our home, which provided a home delivery service. The store was small enough to allow me the opportunity to establish a good working relationship with the pharmacist. There were many times I needed his advice on Larry's care supplies and I appreciated being able to telephone someone who knew me and was familiar with Larry's case. The cost of this service was slightly higher, but I felt it was worth the additional charge. I considered the pharmacist as a very important part of our support team.

Some states have laws that require pharmacists to advise and counsel buyers on how to properly take medications as well as any special instructions, such as not to drink alcoholic beverages, or even milk with some medications. If you have any questions about a drug or any specific instructions, ask the pharmacist. He is a professional and is there to help you.

3. Arrange for Nursing Care

Home care should not be started without the help and advice of a professional nurse, even if it is only for advice at the beginning of home care. Both the doctor and nurse are needed to supervise home care and it is important to set up an initial program of good nursing. The more serious the illness or injury, the more important it is to get professional advice.

Nurses have various levels of education and experience: a registered nurse (R.N.) completes two years minimum academic training to be licensed by the state Board of Nursing Examiners, and many nurses complete higher education courses up to five years. Licensed vocational or practical nurses (L.V.N. or L.P.N.) complete a one year course of academic study to be licensed by the state Board of Licensed Vocational Nurses. The training and requirements for Nurse's Aids varies from state to state. Nurse's Aids obtain approximately six to twelve weeks of training at present. Home Health Aids are usually screened by their experience and provide cooking, housekeeping and minimum personal care. They are not required to have any academic training. Terminology varies from agency to agency and it is best to check academic training and license requirements in your area.

The cost of nursing care is based on the category of nurse. Registered nurses are the highest paid. Nurse's Aids, Practical Nurses and Home Health Aids have a lower rate. The rates per hour vary with geographical area.

The doctor may advise you about the type of nursing care you will need. You will also need a prescription for nursing care as most insurance companies require it to validate claims. Getting it ahead of time will save you having to contact the doctor another time.

HOW TO FIND A NURSE

In the yellow pages of your telephone directory, under the heading "Nurses," you will find several kinds of nursing agencies and registries (operated for profit) and nonprofit agencies which are established to support home care. Commercial agencies operate like other temporary employment agencies. Nursing agencies screen their applicants as do employment agencies of other types, and provide you with referrals of nurses with the skills you need.

Professional nursing agencies (listed as such in the telephone book ads) stipulate that their nurses are members of the state and national nurses' associations. They guarantee that their nurses are thoroughly trained and they require annual physical examinations to assure that the nurses are in good health. Both commercial and professional agencies provide twenty-four hour telephone service.

An example of a nonprofit agency might be your local Visiting Nurse Association. They provide evaluation services and part time nursing care. They also have a twenty-four hour telephone service in case of emergency. Some have sliding scale fees. If you cannot afford nursing care, either through your own resources or insurance coverage, contact your county social service department. Public health nursing visits may be available to you.

Some agencies provide specialized home care services and you will find these listed under home care in your telephone directory.

More and more agencies now support home care and you should be able to locate assistance in your area. If, however, you are unsuccessful in finding a nurse on your own or need advice, you might call your hospital discharge planner for referral and advice.

HOW DO YOU HIRE A NURSE

My first experience in hiring a nurse happened quite suddenly. Larry had come home from the hospital and was not only able to care for himself while I worked, but insisted that he wanted to be independent.

Although I worried a little, I had been advised by the doctor and staff at the rehabilitation unit of the hospital that it was very important for Larry to do as much for himself as he could. So, I repressed my "mother hen" tendency and went off to work leaving him alone in the house, and, after a few days I began to relax and actually enjoyed seeing Larry being self-sufficient again. Then one of Larry's medications was changed. After taking the first pill one evening he became nauseated. In the morning he was still too ill to be left alone, so I phoned nurses' registry, picking one at random. A nurse soon arrived and I went to work.

Larry's nausea subsided after the medication was discontinued but the nurse stayed on for a few days until he could regain his strength. We were both satisfied with this temporary service.

Larry again took care of himself, but occasionally we needed a nurse for a day or two. Then I simply called the agency and they sent someone out. Sometimes we would have three different nurses on three successive days but that did not matter because we knew that it was a temporary arrangement and weren't concerned with establishing a significant relationship.

After one difficult hospital confinement, I realized that we would need a full-time, permanent registered nurse when he came home. From my observation of the several nurses we had worked with I had learned that although they might be equally qualified, there was a vast difference in personalities that affected their abilities to care for specific patients. On a full-time basis these differences could be crucial.

The selection of a full-time registered nurse is not a matter that can be left entirely in the hands of the agency. Only a family member can do final screening that will determine which nurse can best supply not only expert nursing care but can fill the patient's emotional needs as well. Only the right nurse could become a part of our all-important home care team.

Not all nurses are willing to take terminal cases; others aren't able to handle paralyzed patients; some prefer not to work full time or on a long-term basis.

From the nurses who were referred to us by the agency I quickly ruled out, on the first phone call, even those who didn't want to tie themselves up on a long-term case because I was anxious to provide a continuity of care. I also crossed off the list those who began the interview with a list of things they would not do.

That screening left me with but two applicants who came for a personal interview, the means I had decided was essential for making the right choice. One, young and given to nervous mannerisms, talked unceasingly, mostly about her boyfriend. The other, a woman retired from hospital nursing, seemed tired and old, in attitude at least. The first would have been an irritation to Larry, the second could not have given him the confidence and enthusiasm he needed.

When I exhausted the agency's roster, I tried another agency. I was asked to describe, exactly, what I was looking for. I wasn't able to, but I knew I'd recognize the qualities I was looking for when I met the right nurse. But time was running out.

It was Discharge Date Minus Two. Still no nurse and I was worried and was trying to conceal it. Larry had great confidence in me but I knew he was worried about the release date being delayed if we could not find a nurse. Then I got a telephone call from a nurse looking for work. I arranged to meet her at the hospital so that I could combine an interview with an opportunity for her to meet Larry if I thought she was suitable.

She passed her first test when she walked into the room. She was smiling broadly, radiating cheerfulness from every pore. We could use that.

Over coffee in the cafeteria we settled into a serious discussion. As usual, I started with the hardest part.

"Larry is paraplegic. Right now he is bedridden most of the time, but I want to try to get him up in a wheelchair soon, and maybe back on his feet again. This will mean you'll have to learn how to help him from bed to wheelchair. He knows the procedure. I can handle him alone—I was trained at the rehabilitation unit—so I can teach you.

She listened calmly. "Was he in an accident?"

"No," I replied. "He's had cancer for four years. He's back in the hospital because medication given to reduce swelling in the spinal cord caused him to go into a diabetic coma."

We discussed his medical history. I told her a lot about Larry, his interests, background, how we met, our family. I told her that he had been in charge of his care throughout his illness, making decisions, trying to lead as normal a life as possible and to help us all to carry on a normal family life.

I knew she understood that we were looking for a nurse who would virtually become a member of the family, one who would help us make Larry happy and comfortable, one who could delay the morning bath until two o'clock in the afternoon if Larry wanted without flipping her cap.

"I'm not taking him home to die," I told her. "I'm taking him home to live—as well as he can, for as long as he can."

"Larry has what is considered a terminal illness, but I feel he is doing well and has a great deal of courage and a strong desire to live. I want a nurse who will reflect my own optimism, one who will work hard to help him make it."

She didn't flinch from "terminal." It seemed a challenge to her.

Back in Larry's room, she moved a chair close to the bed, sat down and chatted. I was not surprised to hear them laughing a few minutes later. Our search for a nurse had ended.

Later I gave her a tour of our home. Since we had been doing home care previously, everything was set up, but she needed to know where everything was located so that Larry's transition from hospital to home would not interrupt his treatment or care.

If you are doing home care for the first time, the nurse can help you evaluate and prepare the home, advise you on supplies and set up an organized program that will run smoothly and will not require drastic changes once the patient is home.

4. *Arrange for a Physical/Occupational Therapist*

The next member of the home-care team you need to select is a therapist. You will need the advice and approval of a doctor and, again, his written prescription. Some patients may be referred to the physical therapy department of a local hospital on an out-patient basis. If your patient is not able to go to the hospital for therapy, the doctor may recommend a therapist who does home care. If not, you may ask the discharge planner for advice or contact the physical therapy department of a local hospital for referrals. You may also look in the telephone directory (under "Physical Therapy" in the yellow pages) for listings of therapists in your area. If the therapist you call does not do home care, ask him to recommend someone who does or to give you the telephone number of the state American Physical Therapy Association, whose office is usually located in the state capital. The association has a complete list of therapists and will be able to make referrals for home care.

Not all doctors are enthusiastic about physical therapy. They may view the patient's physical condition as irreversible and may feel that therapy is useless. While there may be cases where the injury is permanent, my experience with Larry showed there are no "hopeless" cases. We found that even if one area of the body was disabled, physical therapy strengthened and allowed other parts to compensate. Also, physical therapy provided an emotional stimulation that Larry needed. Just the act of hiring a therapist sent out a clear message: I did not think Larry was hopelessly bedridden, giving him a psychological boost that mere words could never have conveyed.

Some doctors do get locked into the physical diagnosis and do not consider the emotional factors of care. If they will not prescribe a physical therapist and you have decided on physical therapy as a part of the home care you want, I suggest that you consult another doctor.

One of the most important contributions a physical/occupational therapist can make is to evaluate the home and set up a program for patient care which will make the patient more comfortable and easier to care for.

5. *Getting the Home Ready*

Arrange for the physical therapist and the nurse to visit the patient in the hospital to assess his needs and then meet with the family in the home to evaluate and recommend any changes essential for the patient's care.

Safety is of utmost importance. Statistics show that more accidents happen at home than any other place. One very important area of patient care is the bathroom. To avoid falls and accidents, ask the therapist to advise you on how to make your bathroom safe. The two areas of most concern are near the bathtub and shower and around the toilet.

Patients have a tendency to use towel racks, rods, hooks or any other available fixtures to help lift or steady themselves in the bathroom. This is very dangerous because the fixtures are not installed to withstand heavy weight or pressure. If they should pull out of the wall the patient could be injured. Special rods and bars should be installed for the patient's use. Do not purchase these and install them yourself! Get the physical therapist's advice on which rods and bars to purchase (there are many kinds and they can be purchased in various lengths) and at what height and angle they should be installed. Our therapist advised that the rods should be installed by a professional carpenter or plumber whose knowledge of the walls and the studs and pipes behind them would ensure proper and safe installation and might prevent serious injury to the patient.

Remember, the safety and well-being of your patient must be your principal concern.

Some other equipment the therapist may suggest for the bathroom might be: a raised toilet seat or stationary bars around the toilet to assist the patient. Placement of the bars will be determined by the location of the fixtures in the bathroom and the patient's physical problems. The therapist will advise you on whether this should be done before the patient returns home and be ready for use on the first day or if the patient is needed at home first to measure for use.

Some furniture may have to be removed from a room if a hospital bed is needed. Furniture may also have to be rearranged to allow for the use of a walker or wheelchair. Halls and passageways should be free of unnecessary furniture to allow easy access. A bookcase along a hallway wall may look pleasing but may be a hazard if the patient needs to use that hallway to get from the bedroom to bathroom. Footstools or ottomans can be a danger if there is not enough open space in a room, and the patient must go through a maze of furniture to get from one area to another. These footstools are usually pushed away from the chair and may not always be in the same place. Patients may easily trip and fall if furniture is out of place.

Floors should be kept clean, but waxed only if the surface is not slippery. Throw rugs are particularly dangerous. They could slide out from under the feet or trip the patient. Heavy carpeting can make wheelchair and patient mobility difficult. The therapist can train the patient to compensate for this kind of surface, or plastic runners can be tacked down in heavily used areas.

If a patient cannot manage steps or stairs, ramps can be built for easier entry or exit. Ramps can be removable, but it is essential that they be attached to walls or floors when in use.

Other changes may need to be made after the patient is at home, but the major adjustments and installations for safe care should be completed before he arrives.

The therapist will visit the patient either on the day of release or the following day. Frequency of visits will depend on the patient's needs.

6. Purchase Care Supplies and Procure Equipment

The doctor will have indicated on his written instructions the care supplies you will need, or the nurse will have made a list in preparation for home care. Some general items that are helpful to have on hand are:

bandages and gauze pads
tape
thermometers (rectal and oral)
rubbing alcohol
ointment (bacterostatic)
cotton balls and cotton swabs
hydrogen peroxide
oral laxative
rubber or plastic sterile gloves
heating pad
ice bag
facial tissues
soap or lotion (for bathing if skin is dry and sensitive)
hand cleaner (antibacterial)

Always be sure to keep an adequate supply of items available. It is often difficult to get out and purchase items if you should run out. To prevent being inconvenienced, I kept a supply of two of every item on hand.

After you have consulted with the doctor, nurse and physical therapist, you will know what equipment you will need at home to continue care the hospital has been providing. Major items might be:

hospital bed
wheelchair
walker
crutches
portable commode chair
trapeze bar

In order to decide whether to rent, buy or borrow these items you should determine whether you will use the equipment for only a short period of time or on a long-term, permanent basis. For instance, suppose your patient has been in an accident and will be using crutches or a walker temporarily. It would be wiser to borrow them from a local agency. But if you will need a wheelchair permanentaly, you may consider a one-time investment, which is less expensive than renting for a long time.

If you do plan to buy a wheelchair, ask the physical therapist to measure the patient for proper size and adaptations such as length of the foot rests. If a physical therapist is not available, a representative of a hospital supply company can measure for you and suggest adaptations. I strongly suggest that you consider a chair with removable arm rests, to facilitate transferring the patient to and from bed or into a car.

Renting equipment not available from other sources is another alternative. You can select specific equipment and arrange monthly rental payments. This cost is usually covered in your hospital insurance plan if you receive written verification from the doctor.

Borrowing things you need is obviously the best solution. Check with local agencies by telephone to see if they have the items you need. They also provide other services with which you should be familiar. Discharge planners can also refer you to the proper agencies.

If the agencies do not have equipment to loan you, ask if they can arrange discounts on purchase price of special items. Arranging a discount must be done in advance, so don't wait until the day before your patient is ready to go home to do this.

You may also have to be creative and inventive.

We found we could not rent, borrow or buy some apparatus for Larry's care. Larry was a big man. I would have had trouble enough moving him in bed or getting him into a sitting position if he had not required careful handling because of two spinal surgeries. I talked with our sons, Steve and John, about this problem. They designed and were able to build the equipment we needed. We now have a patent on a patient lift board and hope to make the boards available to others who need them.

7. The Patient Care Chart—Write It Down

When you are caring for a patient at home it is *very important* that you have a chart. This not only serves as a reminder on treatment needed but it is also an accurate daily record of patient care. The chart should be prepared while the patient is still in the hospital as soon as the doctor gives you the orders. All information about required care and medication must be on the chart.

You can type an original and then have photocopies made. I suggest you do only about seven copies at first. After your patient has been at home for a week, review the form, make any necessary changes and then have enough copies made in advance to last three to six months. Remember that the chart is made to record daily treatment and medication. As these change, so does the form.

Nursing, cooking, housecleaning, caring for others in the family, are all busy jobs. When you do home care you will find you are jumping from one job to another, and interruptions will become a way of life. You cannot rely on your memory! Don't try. All care and especially medication, must be given as often as directed, in exactly the dosage prescribed and according to all special instructions. Having a chart, controlling and recording care, will be your best aid, your memory bank.

You will learn to check the chart often and after a few days you will have a routine established. Having a chart helps to remind you to get your nursing chores done on schedule.

The chart will enable one person to care for the patient and for another person to come in and know exactly what medication has been given. It is a complete record of care, and is essential for the doctor when he visits.

We used a loose leaf notebook to hold the charts. The doctor's instructions were placed on the left hand inner cover of the notebook. The charts were hole punched and placed on the right hand side of the notebook.

Our charting was done from midnight to midnight, when the date which is on the chart, changes. Our day began at 12:01 a.m. and any charting done after midnight was considered a new day. Since a supply of the sheets was made up and available, anything charted in the early morning hours was put on a new page.

The following is a completed page (illustration A) from the notebook we kept for Larry's care. It is included only as a sample. You will also find a blank form (illustration B) that you may use as a guide to make your own chart to fit your particular needs.

The important items to include are:

Patient's Name

Day of the week: in the event that you do not enter the correct date, you can double check by looking at the day of the week. The day of the week is also a reminder for you, if the therapist visits only on Wednesdays, and you write Wednesday on the chart, it will serve to remind you of the visit.

The date: include the year. Many patients having long-term care will need to keep separate records for each year.

Make a complete list of all medications to be given on the left hand margin of the page. In parentheses list the number of times per day medication is given, dosage and any special instructions. Leave at least three spaces between each medication listed, leaving room to fill in the actual times given.

Physical therapy or exercise: record therapist's visit here.

Temperature: take and record once a day, unless doctor or nurse requests it be taken oftener. If you suspect that the patient has a temperature elevation, you may, of course, take it at any time. If a higher than normal temperature is found, you will want to check it at least every four hours until it returns to normal.

DAILY CARE CHART

For _Larry Baulch_   Date _Thurs._ _June_ _3_ _1976_
                                              Day   Month   Date   Year

MEDICATIONS:

Combid: (one tablet two times per day—
before lunch and dinner)   _11:30 a_   _5:45 p_

Dexymyl: (one tablet four times per
day—8, 12, 4, 8)   _8 a_ _2:30 p_ _4:15 p_ _8:40 p_

Provera: (five tablets three times per
day)   _10:10 a_   _2:30 p_   _10 pm_

Prednisone: (one tablet before breakfast) _7:30 a_

Vitamins: multi, B, C, E, minerals   _9 a_

Demerol: (every four hours as needed   _Dem 50 mg 10 p shot_
Percodan: for pain)   _Perc 5:40 a_   _10:45 a_   _4 p_

TREATMENTS

Sugar test: _Neg_   Morning
                Neg   Afternoon

    Compress solution 4 p, 9:30 p

PHYSICAL THERAPY   ACTIVITY

Mary Kirkpatrick 11 a.m. (1 hr.)   _Up on Wedge 2½ hr._
                                    At dinner time 6:30 - 9 p.

                                      COMMENTS

Bath _10:30 a_   _Blisters appeared with redness_
                            under left upper arm
Diet _Reg_   _Called Dr._
                            Dr. visited at 1 pm
B.M. _10 a Good_   _Diagnosed shingles_
                           New Order —
Liquid input _1900_   _Domebord Powder/Solution_
                    Cool wet compress 4 times daily
Urine output _1400_
          _10 pm_
Temperature _8a 98°_   _Visitor_   _8-9 p_   _Jack, discussed_
                                photography, planned
Blood pressure _100/77_   _an article with Larry_
                                writing/Jack's photos.

(Illustration A)

DAILY CARE CHART

For_____   Date _____
                                      Day   Month   Date   Year

MEDICATIONS:

TREATMENTS

PHYSICAL THERAPY   **ACTIVITY**

                                        COMMENTS

Bath_____

Diet_____

B.M. _____

Liquid input _____

Urine output _____

Temperature _____

Blood pressure _____

(Illustration B)

Blood Pressure: take and record once a day,
unless doctor or nurse requests it
be taken oftener.

List any special care your patient needs daily.

At the bottom of the sheet you can list anything of importance such as bowel movements, catheter care, doctor's visits, any change in status such as "rash appeared—and treatment," nausea, fever, etc. This chart can be made to cover your patient's care and will be specific to his needs.

8. Begin to take home everything the patient will not need again in the hospital.

9. Make arrangements for patient's transportation.

HOMEWARD BOUND

By the time you have completed these arrangements your Home Care Team has been organized. Each of its members—doctor, nurse, therapist, family, pharmacist, yourself and above all, the patient—has a specific role, with responsibilities in the different aspects of the task at hand.

Knowing this will give you confidence, if you are having a few qualms (and you probably are) about your ability to handle the job. The homecoming will be different for every patient and for the patient's family.

This particular homecoming was different for us from others we'd had. I was not having any doubts, but our doctor was. The hospital stay itself had been different.

This time Larry was dangerously ill. He went from one problem to another. He developed a breathing problem and then he got a bladder infection.

This caused an additional three weeks stay in the hospital while he was treated with massive doses of antibiotics and then his blood tests revealed low red cell count. Treatments had helped some, the infection was clearing and I completed our arrangements for going home.

The day before his release I waited with some apprehension for the results of the latest blood test and a meeting with the doctor. His grim face when he entered the room confirmed my anxiety.

The blood count was still low. It might go lower. "Larry may have to come back next week for blood transfusions," he told me.

"I know," I replied, my mind on the four-week hospitalization that, in itself, had become for Larry another one of his problems. I knew the doctor was thinking of our welfare, that I worked full time and couldn't afford round-the-clock nursing care, that I would have to care for Larry two shifts a day weekdays, three on weekends.

But what he didn't know was how much I wanted Larry home and how much I needed him, that I was aware of the amount of hard work and welcomed it just to have Larry home for my sake and for his. This particular hospital stay had been difficult for Larry. He had become discouraged and depressed and I hoped that just being in his own environment, among people who loved him and with the things he enjoyed about him might perform some minor miracle and make him better.

Or maybe he did know, as I knew, just how precarious Larry's condition was, because without a word he signed the release slip. His face was still grim.

Chapter V

Home Care

THE HOMECOMING

Larry was coming home. Despite his worsening condition and the prospect of the additional care he would now require, I was so eager for his homecoming that I set the alarm one hour earlier. I wanted to do a bit of my neglected housework, particularly the bedroom. I put fresh linen on the bed, fresh flowers on the dresser. His favorite food was in the refrigerator.

At no time during Larry's illness did I deny or refuse to accept its realities. But the label "terminally ill" had no application today. I was not bringing him home to die, but to help him live as well as he could, for as long as he could. I felt I could do that at home with the help of my team, better than the staff in the best hospital.

I had arranged with Lyn, his nurse, to go to the hospital and be with him at discharge time. I had spoken with the cashier the day before and completed all financial arrangements. The doctor signed the release form the night before. I had taken home almost all of Larry's belongings and Lyn would have packed up all the remaining things this morning. I had arranged for the ambulance and for Lyn to call me at the office when they left the hospital.

I was always excited about Larry's return home and I waited for Lyn's call with nervous, joyful anticipation. My office was close to home and I arrived well in advance of the ambulance. I opened the garage door so the attendants could bring Larry into the apartment via the ramp. I checked the rest of the house while I waited.

The kitchen was clean because I hadn't eaten any meals at home since Larry went into the hospital three weeks before. The few cups and glasses I had used for a quick breakfast before going off to work all those days were neatly stored in the dishwasher, out of sight. I wiped the table and counter tops with a damp cloth as my eyes kept returning to the window to see if the ambulance had arrived.

Maybe we were closer in some ways than most couples. If we were, it probably had something to do with what had happened years ago, some of it even before we met in 1959.

At that time I was a thirty-one year old divorcee with two small children, working hard to put a shattered life back together. I wasn't looking for another man in my life, nor for another marriage. I had just gotten out of my first marriage, and it had been very painful. But the first time I met Larry at a church dinner, I felt a new kind of life, a sense of excitement come in, a kind of expectancy. I had not felt those emotions for a long time.

After we had known each other for a few weeks, Larry shared the story of his own life with me. In his words he was a "three time loser," a man who had served three terms in San Quentin Prison, a man whose childhood and growing-up years had been deplorable.

It was during his third prison term that he had a crisis experience that led to a complete transformation. I had gone through a transformation of my own, so I could understand what he described to me. With the help of Dr. Cecil Osborne, the minister of my church, Larry had been paroled and worked for the church as an "Assistant Janitor." I knew this was a job they created for him; we didn't need an assistant janitor.

Larry shared with me his dream of hoping to attend a seminary and going back to San Quentin to work. Both seemed like impossible dreams at the time. Seminaries were post graduate institutions and Larry had dropped out of school during his sophomore year, and had only managed to complete his high school education while in prison. He was 33, and it didn't seem likely that he could get four years of college and then attend seminary for three more years. San Quentin did not allow ex-prisoners to visit on a regular basis.

Despite these blatant obstacles, Larry was accepted as an auditing student at the Berkeley Baptist Divinity School. The church sponsored him. He completed all the work of the first semester and enrolled as a full-time student. Three years later he was ordained as a minister in the same church.

Chaplain Byron Eshelman knew of Larry's desire to work at San Quentin. Both he and the church enthusiastically supported Larry's dream. Larry was approved as the first ex-prisoner to be allowed to work in the treatment program at San Quentin. True to his first dream, he immediately returned to enter the grey walls where too many of his young years had been spent. He returned many times during the next ten years, and only ceased going when he became paralyzed.

Larry established the first halfway houses for ex-prisoners in California and worked in prisons and with prison ministry groups all over the United States. In 1968, his first book, "Return To The World," was published.

Larry adopted my son, John, and when several years after our marriage he located and made contact with the two children from his previous marriage, we felt our lives had been blessed. His daughter, Linda, was married and lived in California. His son, Stephen, had graduated from high school, and had enlisted in the Army. My daughter, Carol, had also graduated from high school the same June as Stephen. We were a close, supportive family. The strongest morale force in my team.

The first two years after Larry had surgery for the removal of a cancerous tumor in the kidney, he continued to work and enjoy all his outdoor hobbies. He especially liked to hike and backpack and was considered an expert fly fisherman. Then the tumors metastasized into the spine and within nine months he had undergone surgery twice. After the first operation he learned to walk again but shortly after the second, he lost the ability to move his legs and became a paraplegic.

Although this last hospital stay had been most difficult of all and he had had a series of setbacks, he was still fighting for his life and wanted to be home.

My reverie was interrupted by the sound of the ambulance pulling into the driveway. I hurried outside as the attendants pulled the gurney out of the back of the ambulance. Larry's smile as he reached his hand to me conveyed his pleasure at being home.

"Hi, baby!" he said as I walked alongside the stretcher. "Welcome home," I replied.

As the crew moved Larry into bed I greeted Lyn and walked with her into the apartment. I signed the statement for the ambulance service and then hurried in to see Larry. He was lying in bed, looking around the room at all the familiar objects he loved so much—his photographs of the children, our grandson, Nick, and some friends. There were the watercolors and oil paintings of New Orleans that we had collected on two vacation trips, which hung neatly behind the bed, and his large bookcase filled with his own collection of books.

I sat down on the frame of the bed next to him and gave him a big hug and kiss. Lyn came in and began making some notes on the chart. Larry and I chatted for a few minutes before I returned to work and left him in Lyn's care.

Day one of home care had gone smoothly I learned when I arrived home. I looked over the chart and Lyn explained what I would need to do until she arrived the next morning. After she left, Larry and I settled into our normal family routine, grateful for normality.

Home as Home—Not an Extension of the Institution

Although care previously given by the hospital personnel must be continued at home, the home itself should be maintained as a home and not as an extension of the institution.

Rules which were necessary for institutional care are not needed at home. No visiting hours need be maintained. The patient and the family may decide who they want to visit, when it's convenient for guests to come and how long they may stay.

Baths and meals can be scheduled as the patient requests. No menu need be filled out a day in advance, patients can have the food they want and when they want it. Home care provides an opportunity for flexibility in scheduling.

Patients can read, listen to music, or watch television when they want. They can also rest or take a nap when they are tired. If patients normally stay up late at night and sleep in the mornings, home care can be adjusted to allow it. Avid newspaper readers can arrange to have papers delivered either early in the morning or late in the afternoon, as they prefer. Larry always looked forward to reading the morning paper while he ate his breakfast. It was a long-standing habit with him.

The Importance of Privacy

The home is a reflection of the family's personality. It is the one place it can truly be itself—because home affords privacy and safety from criticism. It is important that this privacy be respected by all medical staff entering the home—they are always a guest in the house. This is particularly true for nurses who do full-time care in someone's home. Problems can develop if the family is comfortable with a cluttered existence and the nurse is a compulsive "there's a place for everything and everything should be in its place" person. Or the other extreme, if a family likes neatness and the nurse has a tendency to leave things in a cluttered manner. The nurse must be able to function as a member of the family and should respect the patterns of living they prefer.

The patient should be able to have some time to spend alone, and should have private visits with guests. One nurse we had for a short period of time not only stayed in the room during the visits but dominated the conversation as well. Of course, visits can be temporarily interrupted to give medications at the proper time but the nurse should not stay in the room during the entire visit. It is important for patients to have freedom and privacy to discuss any personal matters they wish with their guests.

One other benefit provided by the privacy of the home is a normal sexual experience. Although nurses who have worked in hospitals tell me that sexual activity does take place in that institutional setting, the home is certainly a preferred location for intimacy. Unless the doctor strictly orders patients to abstain from sexual activity for their own well-being due to an illness or injury, patients can have a sex life in their own environment. Sex is a natural, strong, human emotion and a successful, satisfying relationship can be extremely therapeutic. If sexual experience is prohibited for a brief period of time to allow recovery from an illness, this promise of resuming sexual activity can stimulate the patient to recover quickly.

Patients and families may feel some reluctance to ask the doctor about the advisability of sex during an illness. I strongly suggest that if you have any doubts or questions that you discuss it with the doctor. After all, sex is affected by emotions and any doubts, fears or anxieties you have could interfere with complete fulfillment and a successful sexual experience.

One of the assumptions most people make is that patients are not interested in sex if they are sick or injured. Not totally true. If a patient is vomiting I doubt if he would be immediately interested in sex. However, some patients have told me that their sexual desire was actually stimulated after surgery—or after the discovery of a terminal illness—or after having a "close call" of some sort. One man told me that he and his wife had an active sex life right up until the time she died of cancer, and that home care allowed them the opportunity to be together—sexually, physically, and emotionally—during those last precious days.

Couples who have had a compatible sex life prior to the intrusion of illness will find ways to continue their experience when the patient is at home. If there were sexual problems prior to the illness, home care may not solve those problems but can provide an environment in which they can be resolved. Illness or injury may further complicate the solution of sexual difficulties, but it could also serve as the motivator to seek professional help. Discuss this with your doctor. If he cannot counsel you appropriately, he can refer you to someone who can.

The home provides a normal setting for living. Families can be together in a place they have created, a place filled with personal belongings to which they have become attached, where they feel most comfortable.

THE TEAM EFFORT

The Patient—Always Number One

The most important member of the team is the patient. Illness or injury is a personal experience and all efforts, decisions and support of the team is for the benefit of the patient.

The patient, himself, must participate in every aspect of the process of care. Other members bring their expertise, their care, their concern and their efforts to the situation. Each member makes a significant contribution, and all work together as a team, for a common goal.

Without the cooperation and positive efforts of the patient, the most dedicated work of all the rest of the team would be in vain.

The Rest of the Team

The first part of the team effort was successful. The family unit was reunited, the doctor was on call, and we had a capable, friendly nurse. The next step was to begin the therapy program.

I had arranged for Mary Kirkpatrick, the physical therapist, to come three afternoons a week. I had never given up the idea that Larry would walk again despite the gloomy, but realistic appraisal of some medical staff. I had learned how to do his physical therapy when he was paralyzed the first time. I continued to exercise his legs even after he was paralyzed this time. I felt that physical therapy was important. He needed to strengthen all his muscles which had deteriorated while he was lying in bed at the hospital with little movement. His arms, especially, needed exercise. He needed to use his arms to enable him to get up in the wheelchair again. In fact, he needed strength just to read or feed himself.

Most important, however, was the psychological factor. I would never concede that he was a hopeless paraplegic. I wanted him to have the best life possible, no matter what his condition. Getting him into a wheelchair meant that we could get out of the bedroom, into other parts of our home and outside via the ramp we had built. Eventually, it would enable us to get him into a car, and out for a drive.

I could not imagine Larry being permanently paralyzed. He was so alive, so athletic. I thought of all the times I had watched him; fly fishing, walking up the center of the stream, leaping from rock to rock to get in better position to cast the fly; jogging six miles per day, round and round a local high school track; all the long walks we had taken up old country roads and abandoned trails; back packing up and down hill (mostly up) to get to a mountain stream in search of the elusive golden trout. I thought of all the miles he drove and the traveling he had done in his ministry.

Now we would have to begin therapy again. Larry had been paralyzed once and had learned to walk again, so we knew it was possible. And physical therapy played an important part in that goal. Mary, Lyn and I were all resolved to do our part to help Larry be as active as possible, beginning with sitting up. At first he could only sit for short periods of time—progressing to longer periods; next was to get up in the wheelchair, and our long-range goal was to have him walk.

Mary began her regular series of visits and instigated an individual program of therapy that was designed to strengthen Larry's upper torso and arms, and to improve his breathing.

During the first weekend Larry was home, Carol, Steve, Nick and my parents came to visit. Friends telephoned at various times. These calls and visits reestablished relationships interrupted by hospital confinement.

The following week, the doctor made his first house call. He examined Larry, took blood samples and checked our home-care chart. The next day he called to report the results of the blood test; although the red cell count was not yet normal, it had improved since Larry came home. We were greatly relieved that Larry would not have to return to the hospital for blood transfusions.

Our home-care team was operational and functioning well. Larry (the patient and most important member of the team) directed his own care. The doctor had full medical control. Lyn and I shared the nursing duties. Lyn was clearly in charge of all technical nursing. I assisted her with the nursing and acted as family coordinator. Mary supervised the therapy part of care and Lyn and I followed her instructions for therapy on days when she did not visit. Although we had not used his services, the pharmacist was available to provide advice on medications and care supplies. Family and friends gave support for our home-care efforts. Each member was equally important but at times one member might assume more responsibility as circumstances required it. We had great respect for each other and were absolutely united in our dedication to the goal of giving Larry the best care possible.

Goals, Duties and Responsibilities of Each Team Member

The primary responsibility of the doctor is to supervise and oversee all medical care. He is the authority on diagnosis, treatment, and medication. It is essential that the doctor and the patient maintain a good, trusting relationship. Patients need to feel secure in the knowledge that they are getting the best medical information and care possible and that the doctor is available for consultation. The doctor-patient relationship is at the very center of home care.

It was interesting to me to look up the word patient in the *Random House Dictionary of the English Language.*

Patient: 1) a person who is under medical or surgical treatment, 2) person or thing that undergoes some action, 3) sufferer or victim.
I have never liked the word patient for just the very reason the dictionary definition states—that a patient is one who is acted upon and is a sufferer or victim. This implies that the doctor or medical staff have a totally active role in the treatment process and the patient has a totally passive role. In many cases that has been the model of the doctor-patient relationship. I have always found this totally unacceptable because it robs the person of the opportunity to participate in his own illness.

Although I have been healthy myself, I found the passive role not only offensive but inaccurate when members of my family needed treatment. I somehow knew that patients must contribute to the healing process and I encouraged my family to do what they could to promote getting well. When Larry was diagnosed as having cancer we both participated in the decision making process and later in all of the treatment he received. The doctor prescribed physical therapy but it was Larry's cooperation, his effort, his strength and his determination that resulted in his being able to walk again. He needed the advice of the doctor and the assistance of the therapists—but they could not exercise for him. He was compensated for his own effort. All patients will gain most by being an active team participant.

Likewise, doctors can prescribe medication but the patient must follow directions and carefully take all medicine as prescribed in order to get well. I've known many people who either:

1. don't take the medication at all
2. take medication for a day or two and then "forget" to take the remaining doses
3. take medicine all at one time because it's inconvenient to take pills every few hours
4. or obtain medicine from a friend because it has worked well for them.

If you are guilty of doing any of the above, you are mis-using the doctor's advice and endangering yourself by not following the doctor's instructions. Doctors can prescribe—but patients must do their part. Doctors do not have control over patients' behavior.

Doctors may advise you that for your own well-being you should quit smoking, lose weight, have a special diet, refrain entirely from alcoholic beverages (or drink moderately), or that you get more rest or sleep. But only you can take that advice and use it. Doctors cannot do it for you, and you should not expect them to give you some sort of magic formula or pill to cure you when you have been unwilling to take proper care of your own body.

Dr. Tom Ferguson began publishing a medical self-care magazine in 1976. He is a strong advocate of patient education and preventive medicine. Most patients, he observed, have competent physicians. They deal with illness or injury (*illness care,* he calls it) after the fact. Dr. Ferguson is encouraging *health care,* which begins while the patient is well.

If you would be interested in finding out more about Dr. Ferguson or his self-care magazines, you may write—*Medical Self Help* Magazine, P.O. Box 717, Inverness, California, 94937.

In addition to information on self-care, the magazine has reviews of books designed to provide knowledge to make you more resourceful, and listings of self-care medical classes for lay people being taught by doctors and nurses.

In *How To Be Your Own Doctor (Sometimes)* Dr. Keith Sehnert presents his concept of what he calls the "activated patient," a lay person trained in basic clinical skills and capable of participating in the management of his or her own illness. Dr. Sehnert teaches self-care classes as well as presenting his work in written form.

Having already come to my own conclusions about the doctor- patient relationship I was pleased to hear a doctor lecture on the subject. David Levenson, M.D. is in private practice in Internal Medicine and is a Clinical Professor at Stanford Medical Center. During the lecture Dr. Levenson used the blackboard to illustrate two conditions: one he called the disease model—the other the health model.

Dr. Levenson told me he did not invent the chart. He said he read a lot and put many ideas together from memory. I am using the chart with his permission and acknowledge his help in structuring this valuable information.

The following is taken both from my notes at the time of lecture in Spring of 1978 and from an interview I had with Dr. Levenson in his office in October of that year.

In the lecture Dr. Levenson gave an example of using the disease model when a patient goes to the doctor and complains of a sore

Disease Model	Health Model
What's wrong?	What's right?
The doctor is active and gives to the patient from a position above the patient.	The doctor is active. He shares with the patient and he is level with the patient.
The patient is passive, takes from the doctor and is in a position below the doctor.	The patient is active, shares with the doctor, and is level with the doctor.
Patient's will is small.	Patient's will is large.
Patient's responsibility is low.	Patient's responsibility is high.*
Mind and emotion focus is on the negative.	Mind and emotion is positive.
Pathologic orientation with a technical focus.	Humanistic—the focus is Holistic (Body, emotion, mind, will and spirit.)
"You are your disease"	"The patient has an illness"

DOCTOR 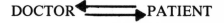 PATIENT

Co-Participants

SICK — UNSICK   WELL

*The doctor takes responsibility for encouraging the patient to become actively involved in his own care. The doctor maintains the responsibility for medical care.

throat. (Disease model—"What's wrong.") The doctor is the active participant and prescribes penicillin. The patient, although cooperating, is primarily in the passive role. The focus is on the sore throat. In this case there is little communication required between the patient and the doctor but the channel is open for feedback if needed. Both the doctor and the patient expect the penicillin to cure the sore throat in a few days.

Surgery as a therapeutic technique for appendicitis also falls in the disease model. Surgery will return the patient to his or her normal lifestyle. The sore throat and the surgery may force patients to convey how they feel and to be in touch with their body functioning but there is no great necessity for strong patient participation.

Dr. Levenson explained, "The patient feels it's here, it's annoying, it's temporary and treatment will take care of it. But chronic illness is one in which essentially there is no penicillin to take care of it, there is no therapy that will make things like new in an acute setting, and very often there is no therapy of the traditional type which comes in to you from the outside and gets you better, i.e. penicillin, physical therapy, surgery. The focus and reality (with chronic disease) is that outside therapy may not be stopping the progression of the illness. That means you are stuck in a place you don't like— like arthritis pain that is killing you all the time—it's not getting worse but you are stuck at that level. I have to do something to help myself to *feel* better in addition to what the doctor is providing me.'"

At this point I asked Dr. Levenson if by "feel better" he meant emotionally.

"Yes. The general quality of life is better. My joints are still painful but I'm doing more and enjoying more. It's quality—it may be on a simple feeling level but it may be on a spiritual level, and it might be on a mental level—I can think more clearly despite the pain in my hands. I can get better in other facets of my life even if my body is not better," he replied.

The disease model on the left side of the board reminded me of a statement I had read in an article on holistic medicine. Dr. Harold Bloomfield, a San Diego psychiatrist said, "People are going to have to take charge of their own health. The reason is that there is something missing in the modern mechanistic view of medicine. You can't always go to the doctor and say 'fix it.'"

I could see the comparison of Dr. Levenson's disease model with Dr. Bloomfield's "Fix it, doctor" approach.

Dr. Levenson continued, "Asthma is reversible, headaches are totally reversible. You could go from one hundred a year to zero. The potential is there. But some things are irreversible—unchangeable. A spinal cord severed by a telephone pole in an automobile accident is irreversible—that will not change. Amputation of limbs—they will not come back. In our society we tend to think if your body isn't good you must feel bad and if you get your body better you will automatically feel good. Of course it doesn't work that way in either direction. That brings up the patient getting involved and the doctor taking responsibility for encouraging that (health model)."

In the lecture Dr. Levenson wrote *Sick-Unsick* under the disease model and *Well* under the health model. The emphasis in the disease model is to be unsick. In chronic illnesses patients may never be unsick (in the physical sense) but they can be well in terms of emotional, mental and spiritual health. I had long believed that the transcendent state of being well has nothing at all to do with the state of the physical body, as in Larry's illness.

In the health model the emphasis is on *what's right.* For instance, if a patient has lost a leg due to an injury, he can become depressed if he centers his attention on the missing part. It is far better to change the focus to emphasize the remaining leg, two arms, eyes that see, ears that hear, voice to communicate, mind that's alert—taking a positive approach to what's right. The patient is active and responsible in the health model and the patient affirms that: "I have an illness or injury," rather than "I am my disease" as in the disease model. The doctor and the patient are coparticipants in treatment in the health model.

In home care it is important that the health model be used and that you become coparticipants with the doctor, not only for your own well-being but for the doctor's. Doctors are human beings and subject to the same stress and illness as the patients. If the doctor has to practice with fifty patients all wanting to operate in the "fix it" disease model, all the strain will be on the doctor. Doctors practice under severe stress and they need all the help, cooperation and understanding they can get. If more patients take responsibility for their own illnesses, the less stress is piled on doctors, allowing them to function better in their professions.

We also need to remember that doctors are human beings—subject to the same emotions, the same joys and sorrows, the same illnesses and health, the same stress, and the physical possibility of death at any time—as are the rest of us. They are not immune to life—but are a part of it.

The primary role of the patient then is to take responsibility for his own health—communicating his ideas, feelings and physical symptoms—and cooperating with medical staff and family.

The nurse's role in treatment is to provide aggressive, solid nursing care for the patient. She must supervise treatment in the home according to the doctor's instructions. She should advise the doctor of any changes in the patient's status and translate his instructions into treatment. She should support and train the family in proper care.

The therapist provides physical rehabilitation and advice, support for total treatment, and emotional stimulation for the patient. She should train the nurse and the family in exercise procedures to give continuity of therapy.

The family and friends provide emotional strength for the patient. Although not all family members and friends contribute to physical care they do provide an important service by their concern. Visits can link a homebound patient to the outside world and broaden the area of interest and associations.

THERAPY

More than anything else it is important to strive to treat your patient as you did before she became ill. Indicate by your attitude that you expect her to recover, that she is still a part of the family.

Allow her to do everything that she can do for herself, encourage her to share her feelings—good and bad—and to participate in plans for the future.

By taking her home you have removed her from the hospital (i.e. sick) setting. Continue in that direction. Unless she is a complete bed patient, urge her to get dressed. Pajamas, bathrobe and slippers are appropriate in a hospital, but getting dressed and groomed affirms normal living. Loose fitting, comfortable, easy-care clothing may be needed if the patient has bowel or bladder problems.

Therapy is the first step back to normal living. The physical therapist can provide a great many benefits and should be a part of your team even if your patient is elderly or terminally ill. The former patient needs the treatment to prevent further deterioration; the latter for the psychological lift and sense of hope it contributes.

My enthusiasm for therapy comes from the benefits Larry and I received from therapists' professional care and positive attitude.

When Larry was paralyzed the first time, the paralysis came suddenly. Neither of us knew anything about physical handicaps. Larry had surgery immediately after a tumor that pressed on the spinal cord was discovered. I sat and waited, thinking about the surgeon's words. "We'll do what we can but there is no guarantee he'll regain his ability to walk. He may be a permanent paraplegic."

The doctor came to the waiting room after surgery. "I removed as much of the tumor as I could to relieve the pressure on the spinal cord. We will have to discuss getting some radiation therapy to deal with the remaining tumor."

"Will he walk again?" I asked.

"We won't know that until tomorrow. He's too sleepy from the anesthesia to respond tonight," he replied.

I saw Larry briefly that night. He was amazingly alert. He smiled at me and I held his hand and kissed his forehead. As I drove home I was thankful that we knew the cause of the paralysis, that the surgery was over and Larry was alive. I wondered what the next day would bring . . . but the joy and relief I felt far outweighed any anxiety.

The next morning I was awakened by the sound of the telephone ringing. I picked it up with the fear that this might be some kind of emergency. Nobody ever calls to give you good news at this early hour!

"This is your husband's nurse in the intensive care unit," she said. "Your husband wants to know when you're coming to see him." I smiled the smile that comes from knowing the one you love loves you. I settled back on the pillows and relaxed, feeling the tension released. "When can I visit?" I asked.

"You can come anytime you want, but the length of time you stay is limited."

"Tell him I'll be there as fast as I can . . . and that I said thanks for waking me up."

By the time I arrived Larry had eaten a breakfast of bacon and eggs and he was ready to talk. "I have a surprise for you," he announced proudly. "Lift up the sheet at the foot of the bed." I lifted it up and he moved his big toe. It was the most beautiful sight I had ever seen!

Larry was transferred from the intensive care unit to a private room. We began six weeks of radiation therapy on the remaining tumor and he had limited physical therapy while he was in bed. I watched the therapist and repeated the exercises with Larry each evening and on weekends.

When he was released from that hospital, he was admitted directly to a rehabilitation spinal cord disability unit in a hospital about fifty miles from our home. The doctor arranged to have him transported by ambulance while I was at work. I went down immediately after leaving my job. Larry was sitting in his wheelchair by the front door when I pulled up in the driveway, stopped and blew the horn. He smiled and waved enthusiastically. I drove off to find a parking place, then ran back to be with him.

It was the first time I had seen him dressed since his surgery. He told me he had dressed himself lying in bed—no small chore. He took me on a tour of the department. His room was a four-bed ward. None of the other three patients spoke English but we waved to them as we came into the room. Above each bed was a chart marked *I DID THIS FOR MYSELF TODAY,* under which was a double list of things to be checked off. Patients were not only encouraged but expected to do everything for themselves they could. There was a dining room-recreation room equipped with TV and wheelchair-high pool table. The physical therapy area was larger than any I'd seen and there was a swimming pool, also for therapy. The staff was friendly and they were obviously dedicated to this rehabilitation work.

Rehab therapy was an all-day, continuing process. No one-hour sessions in this department like the other hospital. The staff was helpful and eager to teach me how to help Larry. Families were considered a part of the team. The whole operation was geared to get the patient home and to make him as independent as he could be. I discovered in my first conversation with the therapist that they did not "feel sorry" for the patient. Pity is a poor basis for restoring independence and motivating patients to do more. Staff members were ready to be supportive, but they forced the patients to try everything themselves. If he failed, the staff explained what went wrong and encouraged him to try again and again and again until he achieved the success he was striving for. Then a big check mark was posted on the board and everyone was genuinely pleased to see the progress.

One night that first week the nurse greeted me with a "snicker" when I walked in. "Your husband has something funny to tell you tonight. Ask him about his therapy today." Larry was already in the dining room having dinner when I arrived in the unit. I sat next to him as he ate and then we went for a walk. He maneuvered the wheelchair down the hallway into a quiet area. My motherly instinct wanted to help him but I had learned the therapist's lesson well and knew he had to do it himself. If he tired, we simply stopped and rested.

"What funny thing happened in therapy today?" I asked. Larry broke out in laughter and told me that he had gotten out of the chair and was practicing walking between two parallel bars, which he held with both hands to keep the weight off his legs. He said he was concentrating and working with great effort to get the legs to move, one in front of the other. The therapist was in front of him giving verbal directions, when his pants slipped from around his waist and fell around his ankles! There was no way he could let go of the bars to pull them up himself. Everyone began to laugh—most of all Larry and the therapist. She simply leaned over, pulled up the pants and got a piece of rope to use for a belt to hold them up. "Maybe you can bring me a belt," he suggested.

I appreciated his sharing the story and I was glad he had people working with him who had a good sense of humor.

Larry liked the pool therapy. He could move easily in the water. He was a good swimmer and the water held up the weight of his body so he could exercise his legs without fear of falling. His legs grew steadily stronger and he was getting more check marks on the chart.

I was awed by our feeling that we were lucky he had only lost the use of his legs. Good strong arms are a real asset in this department. Some patients did not have any use of their arms; some had little. Some used wheelchairs with a mouth piece which was used to move the wheelchair. They were the ones who could go the fastest up and down the hall. But regardless of how much or how little they had to work with—the staff brought out the best in every patient. I admired their spirit and I'm sure that part of my own attitude about Larry's new life was formed there.

At the end of three weeks Larry announced that he had passed all of the required tests (including driver's training), proving he was able to go home and take care of himself. But he could not be released until I could come in for a meeting with the staff. They considered me a very important part of the team and I was pleased that I could do something to help. We met that morning with seven staff members.

I had heard about the doctor who headed the department. The lower portion of his body was paralyzed from polio. He ran the department from his wheelchair. The patients looked out the window every morning as he arrived in his specially-equipped car with hand controls. He pulled the wheelchair out from behind the seat, set it up next to the driver's side, and transferred himself into the wheelchair. He then closed and locked the car door and wheeled himself into the building to begin another day of seeing patients. "What an inspiration he must be," I thought.

The staff asked if we had any questions. By this time Larry had already had two "weekend passes," giving us an opportunity to try out what we learned at the hospital. The staff had done their job well and our only questions dealt with continuing care in our home and what recommendations they had for continuing physical therapy. Larry had made amazingly fast progress. He could dress himself, transfer from the bed to wheelchair and back again unaided. He could use the bathroom facilities alone, and was on his feet walking in a walker.

The day before Larry was to be discharged from the rehabilitation unit, he asked me if I could have the Spanish teacher at the school where I work write a message that he could read to his three Spanish speaking roommates. Larry had been in the room over three weeks and verbal communication had been possible only when a Spanish speaking staff member would translate. Larry carefully wrote a short message in English that he wished to convey. The next day when I came to take him home, I brought the Spanish version. Larry read it while sitting in his wheelchair as he was ready to leave. As he read, they began to smile and then to laugh. They were laughing partly at his stumbling pronunciation and partly at the message itself. But it was clear to see they appreciated his efforts. As we passed by on the way to the car they continued to wave and shout greetings through the window.

Larry was able to come home and care for himself. He even wanted to do his own cooking. He was so proud of the fact that he was able to do it and needed no nursing care. The only help he needed at first was being driven to physical therapy. We had a steep driveway and there was no way he could maneuver the wheelchair uphill alone. I called a nearby college and hired a student to come to do this for us. At therapy Larry learned to walk with a cane and climb steps. He also continued swimming therapy to strengthen his legs. At the end of nine months we were again taking long walks together, traveling in the car, and even took a trip by plane to Las Vegas. We rented a car and did a four-day tour of Bryce Canyon and Zion National Park. Our son, John, went with us and this was a memorable sight-seeing trip. It was September and all the world seemed golden.

Physical Therapy

Physical therapy is chiefly geared toward improvement or a return to normal function. It can also be an important factor in creating an atmosphere of constructive effort toward the goal of health in which the patient himself is an active participant.

If your doctor has not ordered physical therapy for your patient you may suggest it. You cannot obtain the services of a physical therapist without a doctor's orders. If damage has been severe or if the patient has had orthopedic surgery, a doctor specializing in physical therapy may be needed to supervise treatment.

Some patients who have begun physical therapy while they were hospitalized may be able to continue therapy on an out-patient basis. They may also be referred to a private physical therapy department or other rehabilitative facility such as Easter Seals. When patients are unable to get out of the home, you can arrange for a therapist to come in by discussing it with your doctor. The physician may recommend a specific frequency of visits and directions for therapy or may order physical therapy with the program being established by the therapist. The patient's financial status may also be a consideration in determining the number of visits.

Home therapists are available in all geographic areas. They can set up a program for patients to follow on their own (with periodic checks by the therapist) or arrange visits to do physical therapy with the patients. In either case, the therapist would give instructions to the family and/or nursing personnel.

What can you expect your physical therapist to do for you? The therapist can:

1. Establish goals of treatment with the patient and family by discussing the patient's present status, expectations of the patient, family and therapist, and ways in which those agreed upon goals can be accomplished.
2. Instruct the patient and family in the use of equipment.
3. Instruct the patient and family in the routine daily functions.
4. Instruct in safety procedures.
5. Instruct the patient and family in an exercise therapy program.
6. Assess pain and provide therapy treatment for relief.
7. Provide a supportive, therapeutic relationship with the patient and family.

At the beginning of home therapy, the patient, the family, and the therapist must agree on reasonable goals for therapy. In order to assure full cooperation between the therapist and family, it is imperative to reach an agreement establishing goals before therapy is begun. This is accomplished by discussing hopes and expectations of what they want to achieve through a therapy program. Everyone needs to express himself fully, thereby opening lines of honest communication. Therapists will be able to advise the patients and families on whether or not their goals are realistic. Therapists have a responsibility to counsel them when their expectations are unrealistic. Once mutual goals have been established, everyone can put full effort into making the therapy successful.

The patient's progress will be evaluated by the therapist at regular intervals to determine if the goals need to be adjusted. Ongoing therapy requires constant reassessment.

Therapists can train the patient and family in the proper use of equipment such as wheelchairs, canes, crutches, and walkers. They also supervise use, checking the height of walkers to be certain the patients can attain the best control and adjusting crutches for axillary armpit position. If crutches are not at the proper height for the individual patient, there will be pressure on the nerves that pass over the axillary area. This pressure can sometimes permanently damage the nerves, resulting in motor and/or sensory loss. Patients are instructed to place their weight on the hand pieces rather than armpit rests.

The physical therapist will observe patients in the home situation and recommend any changes needed to assist the patient's mobility. For example, the therapist can advise the family on installation of a ramp if one is needed. The angle of the ramp must be determined by the amount of disability the patient has. Going up a ramp in a wheelchair demands a great deal of effort. The more disability, the lower the degree of angle of the ramp will need to be. For safety, ramps must be attached to walls and floors and the ramp surface must have either a nonskid covering or have horizontal nonskid strips to prevent slipping. A hand rail is also advisable.

Sometimes illness or injury hamper the patient's ability to function normally in routine daily activities. The physical therapist helps the patient and family adapt and adjust to the situation as it presently exists, teaching them to function as best they can. This includes teaching the patient how to get in and out of bed safely; on and off the toilet; in and out of tub or shower; in and out of a chair; move from room to room, in and out of doors; up and down stairs; in and out of a car. These skills become easier for the patient with practice, and improve the quality of his daily life.

The physical therapist may recommend to the physician that the patient have training by an occupational therapist when such therapy is indicated.

Occupational therapists, also rehabilitative therapists, can train the patient in activities of daily living such as dressing, bathing, grooming, eating, housekeeping activities, and in the use of any adaptive equipment for those skills.

For example, for a stroke patient, with paralysis on one side of the body a physical therapist would set up a program to improve joint motion and muscle strengthening, would instruct the patient in proper ambulation and use of equipment while the occupational therapist would train the patient to dress, groom, and feed himself and in the use of any equipment to accomplish these tasks.

If a stroke patient has the use of only one hand, the occupational therapist can show him how to dress one handed. If the patient has arthritis and loss of hand function, the occupational therapist can suggest adaptive equipment to help him dress, advise using velcro tape on clothes instead of buttons, stocking aids and long-handled shoe horns for help in putting on shoes. Adaptive equipment is also available to assist in eating. If a patient is in a wheelchair all or most of the time, the occupational therapist may recommend some adjustments to keep household items at a level where the person can reach them unaided. For instance:

In the kitchen: Cooking utensils, dishes and food should be within easy reach.

Bathroom: Personal items, towels and wash cloths, toilet paper and soap should be accessible.

In closets: Things should be stored at a median level, not on shelves above clothing hung on rods or on the floor. Storage bins and shoe racks can be purchased in a notions department of most stores. These will enable you to store items so they can be easily retrieved.

In dressers: Top and bottom drawers may not be convenient but the two or three middle drawers usually work well. A little rearranging saves the frustration of having to ask someone to get things that are just out of reach. Patients cannot be totally independent if they do not have easy access to items they need in the process of every day living.

If a patient needs specialized job training to either return to work or find a new occupation, the therapist may refer him to the state Department of Rehabilitation which provides this service.

Physical therapists train patients in safety procedures which is a routine part of therapy. They teach patients the safest ways to use equipment, make transfers, ambulate, fall if they lose their balance, examine themselves for injuries once they've fallen, and get up off the floor. Even if there is a family member to assist, it is important that patients know how to do these things for themselves. It is especially important for persons living alone to learn these safety measures. Family members are trained in proper procedures if the patient needs assistance.

An essential part of a physical therapy program is a plan of exercises to attain the goals established. Therapists set up an exercise program that patients can do themselves or with assistance of family members. In an on-going physical therapy situation, therapists administer specialized exercises with the patients. This program is different from the program set for patients to do themselves. For maximum progress, therapy will include both regular visits with the therapist and patients exercising on their own.

Bed patients particularly need exercise to improve circulation resulting in increased blood flow to prevent phlebitis, which is a major concern. Due to nonactivity, bed patients tend to breathe shallowly, depriving the muscles of needed oxygen. Breathing exercises increase lung capacity (vital) and improve oxygenation of tissues. The goals are to prevent complications, and maintain present level of body functioning, with expectation of improvement.

Pain control and relief are important aspects of the patient's well-being. Pain interferes with daily activities, hampers progress in therapy, and affects personal relationships. A team effort is needed to determine treatment although the physician orders all treatment. Pain control is discussed at length in a later chapter.

Attitude affects physical therapy. If a patient shows initiative, self-motivation, and a positive attitude, his exercise will be done with enthusiasm. The more effort the patient puts into therapy the better the results will be. A patient who says "I'll never be better," or "What's the use?"—reflects a self-defeating attitude, and does not give his full support to therapy. Part of the therapist's job is to encourage the patient to contribute what he can to reach short-term realistic goals.

Rapport between the patient and therapist is an essential ingredient to successful physical therapy. Some therapists suggest that the relationship is even more important than the techniques they use. Patients who trust their therapists will respond willingly to instructions. It is sometimes frightening for patients to try to walk when they have been disabled. Therapy requires repetition of exercises and procedures to strengthen physical weaknesses and develop new skills. Therapy has a natural trial and error aspect and the therapist and family must be patient when goals are not accomplished quickly. The therapist will encourage patients to keep trying and be enthusiastic. If realistic, mutual goals have been set, neither the patient, the family nor the therapist will be disappointed in results. Physical therapy may be a long, continuing process. If the patient and therapist have a good relationship, even extended therapy will be productive, pleasant and enjoyed by all participants.

I noticed the therapists at the rehabilitation unit had a good sense of humor. They did not dwell on the tragically serious nature of an illness or injury. Centering on the loss of function or disability can be depressing to both the patient and staff. Sometimes humor is the only way to ease tension constructively in unusual or difficult situations. If we can laugh at ourselves and our circumstances, they somehow don't seem unbearable.

Fortunately for us, Larry's therapist, Mary Kirkpatrick, had a sense of humor. She and Larry enjoyed their sessions and therapy itself was not the most important consideration. Larry looked forward to her visits and she brought as much enjoyment and happiness into his life as she did professional skill. They shared common interests, and talked about a variety of subjects during the hour she was with him. In addition to her friendliness, Mary was a diligent therapist and could get Larry's cooperation to a greater degree than either Lyn or I could.

The relationship with the therapist provides the patient with another person to talk with and another source of advice. Some patients may share their concerns and fears about recovery more freely with the therapist than with their family. They may not want to worry the family, or they may feel family members cannot answer their questions as well as the therapist.

An acquaintance, whom I will call Jerry, for example, feared he would not be able to successfully complete therapy and eventually return to work. His family, wanting to bolster his courage, talked about "when you return to work," and made statements like, "just keep trying and before long you'll be your old self." Jerry had doubts about his recovery. He wanted the truth and he asked the therapist for her opinion.

The therapist recognized the impasse and stepped in as mediator with Jerry and his family. It turned out that going back to work was a possibility—but not for a long time. This meant the family needed to make financial plans, including applying for long-term aid. In some cases, return to work is a definite option but the patient is not aware of his true progress.

Therapists may help patients view their therapy realistically and reassure them of the successful outcome. The therapist may (with the patient's permission) discuss the problem of communication with the family if they are mistaken in their view of the progress and might discuss the situation with the family and patient together. The therapist can determine the best course of action, always respecting the privacy of the patient. Naturally, if what the patient shares is confidential, the therapist will only listen and advise but not discuss.

If the patient shares a problem that is beyond the scope and knowledge of the therapist, the therapist will suggest a consultation with the doctor, nurse, or social worker. Any assistance the therapist can give to eliminate or handle problems will free the patient for successful physical therapy.

There was the case of Marion, a wheelchair tyrant.

All her life she had waited on and cared for other members of the family.

When she became disabled, she hated being in a wheelchair and when she came home from the hospital, she was full of hostility and resentment for her situation. She turned this on her family and became alternately a martyr (poor me, having to be in this situation while you're all well and having a good time) and a dictator, making needless demands and ordering everyone around.

The family didn't want to add to the woman's already difficult situation. Partly out of guilt for their own wellness, and past favors, they obeyed all her commands. Their compliance robbed her of the opportunity to do things for herself, a healthier option than being waited on constantly.

In a normal family situation, someone would have told her that her demands were dictatorial, and excessive. They might even have refused to comply with her demands. They probably would have yelled back at her when she yelled at them. But her illness put them all in a new situation. There was no therapist to observe both sides of the problem.

One day, a friend of the woman came to visit. She got the tyrant treatment. When Marion made angry demands, the friend calmly and firmly refused. She also told Marion she did not enjoy being treated in such an unkind manner (which was a true statement of her own feelings). She pointed out to the surprised Marion how her attitude affected their friendship. For the first time Marion was made aware of what she had been doing to those around her.

Treat the patient as a normal person. And most importantly, remember that being normal means that both the patient and family have the right and the responsibility to share their feelings. Relationships do not grow out of subterfuge—but out of genuine concern and love for each other.

Speech Therapy

Accidents, degenerative diseases and strokes can affect a patient's speech. The psychological aspect of loss of speech can be more devastating than a physical one. The patient faces two battles—physical disability and psychological disability.

A speech therapist, unlike a physical therapist, does not need an order from your doctor to treat the patient. You may be referred to one by a doctor or other medical staff member, or you may simply contact a therapist for treatment on your own.

The illness or injury that affects the speech may also affect the functioning of the brain where thoughts and feelings are formed. In this case the therapy will need to include, when possible, retraining another part of the brain to do the work previously done by the damaged part, and retraining speech functions to convey the thoughts formed by the brain.

The speech pathologist will diagnose the problem and as with other types of therapists, help patients form reasonable goals and set up an individual program of therapy.

The program will likely include:
1. Strengthening of weakened oral muscles.
2. Retraining the brain patterns to form words and thoughts.
3. Counseling patients and families.
4. Helping patients live as normal a life as possible.

Articulation, the production of speech sounds, may be one problem. A person might develop poor points of articulation as a central nervous system disorder becomes more degenerative. Patients need therapy to form proper speech habits, to restore speech loss or impairment. A hearing loss can affect the normal monitoring system of speech and articulation. Some patients have a weakening of oral musculature and the muscles can be strengthened through therapy. Some patients have paralysis. Others have more severe problems due to the surgical removal of the larynx or other muscles needed for proper speech. Patients sometimes have other physical problems related to speech technique. Salivation and drooling occur when patients cannot keep their lips closed. Problems sometimes interface with reading and language skills. The determination must be made whether the problem is speech technique, brain function, vision or hearing loss, or a combination of these.

Again as with other therapists, the speech pathologist works with the entire family as a unit, counseling each member as needed and serving as an advisor. The family, in turn, is able to furnish helpful information that enables the therapist to evaluate the patient by comparing his former function with present function.

The important thing to remember is that it is not only a matter of how well the patient can verbalize, read or write but how he handles his emotions and how he feels about what has happened to him.

Doctors and therapists explain to patients what has happened to them. The doctors may explain initially and therapists may discuss it again in terms of therapy. But someone needs to communicate somehow with patients—in spite of any handicap they have in communicating—in layman's terms they can understand. A lack of communication can affect all areas of the patients' lives. It begins in the hospital and continues at home unless someone can communicate what is happening.

The patient and family are under a great deal of stress at the time of the illness or injury and they need a calm, assuring attitude on the part of the professionals to avoid misunderstandings. Therapists can act as mediators because they understand the disability of the patients.

Stroke patients sometimes understand the spoken word but cannot express themselves through speech. In some cases they have difficulty understanding the spoken word when sentences or phrases are longer. Very often the stroke patient will have some difficulty in both areas of speech and understanding the spoken word, rather than having difficulty totally in one or the other. Speech therapists have the vast professional knowledge to evaluate, diagnose, and help retrain people with communication difficulty.

The disease or injury determines the amount of impairment or speech loss. Patients' language functioning will be at its worst after a stroke but there is an opportunity to help them live in their new state and there is hope of improvement with therapy. Other degenerative diseases have a slowly worsening pattern. The therapist can teach the patients skills to function as best they can. Some injuries cause damage that is irreparable. Even in these situations, the therapist can help the patient live as fully as possible.

I met with Aline Fisher, a speech pathologist at Letterman Army Medical Center in San Francisco. She was kind and generous in sharing her professional knowledge and experience. She, like so many other professionals I have met, is obviously dedicated to her patients, believes in her work, and cares greatly for people. Aline works not only with active duty and retired military personnel but with their dependents as well. Her past experience includes working in a school system, being an instructor of speech pathology at the college level, and working as supervisor in a speech and hearing clinic. It is important to remember that there is a direct relationship between speaking and hearing. You may need to use two professionals in your therapy—a speech pathologist and an audiologist.

I talked with Aline Fisher about the emotional stress of illness. She said "I think it is important to note that people's personalities are personified when they are ill. Their moods are going to change and even though it is a period of transition, a lot of things are changing at the same time and you just have to go with them. You have to help patients and families express their feelings and not be embar-

rassed by those feelings. It is also important to treat patients as the adults they are and not as children. In other words, don't talk down to a patient but recognize that he is a human being—with an illness or injury that has affected him—and that he is still a person."
Families need to understand what has happened to the patient because they will be playing an important role in therapy.

A patient may suddenly wake up after an accident, or stroke and find he cannot speak—or speak and only make garbled sounds or unintelligible word patterns. He may say things and realize no one can understand him. Patients, such as those who have a laryngectomy, can communicate by writing out their thoughts and feelings. Aline Fisher told me she has patients use either pencil and paper or a "magic slate," a children's toy which has a plastic film over it that can be lifted to quickly erase the writing.

Some patients, such as those having strokes, may even lose the ability to write out messages. But even if the patients cannot communicate with others, they still have a hearing function. Staff and family can speak to them. Even if communication is one sided—it is better than no communication at all.

Sometimes patients come out of a state of unconsciousness with an angry, hostile attitude, hitting at nurses, attempting to pull out IV tubes, throwing things on the floor. This anger, therapists agree, may be rooted in fear and patients need to communicate these feelings.

Patients who are angry and hostile may add to the family's problems unless they have a safe outlet for their emotions. Families and medical staff also need to share their feelings about dealing with this kind of behavior effectively. Group counseling provides a place for this kind of sharing.

When some brain damage has occurred, patients may have a very limited vocabulary, with all or most of it profane. Even with patients who would never use swear words as part of their normal speech (even ministers and nuns), the words may still be spoken. Therapists will try to teach the patients a few basic words like "hello" and "goodbye," but the patients may attempt to say hello and a profane word will take its place. Families need to be aware that this uncontrolled response should not be an embarrassment. Any uncomfortableness or embarrassment felt by family members will be transferred to the patient. Families cannot control speech patterns but therapists can help families to react in a positive emotional way in this situation.

If patients stutter and have difficulty forming correct words, the therapists will help families respond appropriately and can teach families ways to help patients become more successful in speaking.

Family roles and responsibilities sometimes have to be shifted or switched when an illness or injury occurs. Fred, who had worked and supported his family, made decisions for them and was the literal head of the household, suffered a damaging stroke. Ellen, his wife, who was comfortable in a supporting role, had to now make all major decisions, including assuming responsibility for supporting the family.

Jean was on her way to work when she was involved in an auto accident. Serious injuries required a long recuperation period. Her husband, Tom, assumed all household responsibilities and care for the children along with having to adjust the family finances pressured by the cost of care and his wife's lost income.

Such major life changes may require counseling, not only for the patient's recovery and rehabilitation, but for smoother family adjustments as well.

Families must be realistic about what patients can and cannot do and whether the situation is transitional or permanent. Even with a permanent disability there is an opportunity for quality of life.

Laura had always wanted to take art lessons but had not taken the time from family duties to pursue her interest. At age fifty-seven she had a stroke. As part of a long-term therapy program she was required to swim regularly, exercising in a pool. One day she noticed some paintings on display when she went for therapy. She decided that now was her opportunity. She enrolled in art classes, at first doing simple color work, advancing slowly as her function and coordination improved. Her illness provided some free time to do something she had long wanted to do, and the art form gave her a new medium of communication.

Ongoing counseling is an essential part of therapy. Counseling is carried on in a number of ways, individually with the patient and family members, with the family together as a group and with groups made up of husbands of patients, wives of patients and children of all ages. This group counseling enables family members to be aware that they are not the only ones faced with problems— and spouses and patients can effectively counsel one another.

Group counseling and laymen helping laymen are used in many

kinds of organizations. Alcoholics Anonymous has groups for spouses of alcoholics (called Alanon) and groups for children of alcoholics (called Alateen). Many other organizations utilize the collective wisdom and strength of such groups.

Some patients can function in their marital lives after illness or injury—both physically and psychologically—others cannot. Sophie, who spoke both English and a foreign language, was in her eighties when she had a severe stroke. After the stroke, she spoke only in her native tongue. Her husband, who spoke only English, was hard of hearing and communication with staff members was hampered. Sophie remained in the hospital because her husband could not care for her at home. And he, like many men, found it difficult to spend much time visiting her. Their relationship was deteriorating in both the physical closeness and in communication. They grew more and more apart. She died a few months after the stroke.

Norman had a heart attack. A few weeks later, his wife fell and sustained an injury that affected her speech. They began to go away on weekends together to help each other recuperate. Their relationship was enhanced by the adjustments they made.

A man who owned his own business had a stroke. Although he was not capable of running the business afterwards, the wife instructed the employees that he was still the boss and they should do what he told them to—even if it meant they would have to redo the work later to correct his errors. The man went to the office and worked as much as he could, which was only an hour on some days. She also told her husband that they had always made love before the stroke, that they still loved each other, and that she expected him to perform his marital duties for her. She appealed to his sense of self-worth and independence and they worked out a satisfying life despite his illness.

Aline Fisher told me, "If you can't laugh about your own problems then the seriousness will get to you. If you get too serious, especially with an illness, (and Lord knows there is enough to be serious about, you get it from every test and diagnosis,) you lose perspective. It's all very serious and it should be. But I think there has to be a point with either the therapist or in a group counseling situation and certainly in a home setting, that you allow a place for humor."

Speech pathologists, like other therapists, are very supportive of patients and families and make a significant contribution in rehabilitation. You can find them listed in the yellow pages of your telephone book under "Speech Pathologists" or your doctor may refer you to someone. Your county medical association office or hospital discharge planner are other sources.

Speech pathologists are another important part of the team effort.

PHYSICAL CARE OF THE PATIENT

Now that your patient is home, the doctor will order all treatment and prescribe medications, and the nurse and/or family members will provide all physical care. It is important to carefully follow the doctor's instructions and to use the chart to record all care and treatment given.

Physical care is supervised by a nurse. Even if you only have a nurse to provide instructions and set up a program initially or have a regular duty nurse, you will need assistance.

This section on physical care is not meant to be a substitute for professional advice from a nurse. I am not a professional nurse and even though I provided care for Larry and other family members, I do not have the education or experience to advise you on technical nursing. Even if I were a nurse, I would not advise you on care for your patient. There is a risk of misunderstanding in attempting care by merely reading about it. The nurse will advise and train you in the specific skills and knowledge you need in your individual circumstance. For any given situation there may be more than one way to handle care. A nurse familiar with your particular problem can best evaluate and advise you or will consult the doctor, therapist or other professional who can suggest effective care or treatment.

Don't be overwhelmed by your lack of medical knowledge. Rely on your nurse to train you in each function of care needed. It will probably not be necessary to learn all techniques at once. You can learn by assisting the nurse and observing her. The nurse can observe as you learn each process and assist until you both feel confident of your ability to function on your own. Patients often feel confident when you do. And they will let you know if they feel uneasy about any care technique.

If you want to learn more about technical nursing care, the nurse can recommend books on nursing procedures or related topics that you may read to become more knowledgeable. But books should never replace professional training.

Be sure to ask questions about anything you do not understand. Asking questions is not a sign of ignorance but rather the first step to wisdom.

Medication

The administration of medication must be done precisely as ordered by the doctor. The chart is set up to establish a time sequence in which medicines are given. There is little decision making in the medication process. The doctor has already prescribed the drug, the dosage, and the time it should be given. The major responsibility of the nurse and family is to follow orders: to give the exact medication, the correct dosage and at the proper time intervals. Accurate charting is a must for all phases of treatment but particularly for the giving of medication. An important part of the charting procedure is to also note any changes in the patient which may indicate to the physician a need for modification of the patient's prescription.

If you are planning to the take the patient out in the car for a period of time, you will need to plan to take along any medicine to be given during that time. If you are giving drugs in pill form, you will also need to take along (or arrange to get) some liquid and a glass to facilitate pill taking. If you are administering medication in shot form, you will need the syringe, alcohol-soaked cotton pad and band-aid to cover injection site. These, of course, will need to be kept sterile. If you need to give liquid medication, be sure to take along a spoon.

If you are entertaining guests or are having a family celebration, it is easy to lose track of time and get off schedule in giving medicine. It is best if you devise a reminder system such as a note pad posted on the refrigerator door if you are working in the kitchen, setting a timer or clock to go off at the time you need to give medicine, or mentally connecting the time for giving medication with some other event (if you plan to serve dinner at 6:00 P.M. and the patient is due to get a pill at 6:00 you will remember to give the pill before serving dinner).

Find a convenient place to keep *all* medications. If possible, keep the chart and the medication in the same location for accurate charting. Pick a spot in full view; a medicine chest is not a good place because it is not visible. Keeping medications in sight is another good reminder to assure proper administration. Some medications need to be refrigerated. Be sure and read the labels for instructions.

If you have several medications to give it may not be convenient to have them in an area that requires your making repeated trips.

Considering all these points, I decided to keep Larry's supply of medications on the top of a dresser near his bed. The notebook containing the doctor's instructions and chart was also placed on the dresser, opened to the daily log page. The bottles of pills and liquids were placed on a silver tray that we had received for a wedding gift but seldom used previously. It added a nice touch to the room, and was a way to make the pill supply area look more attractive. Using a pill tray permitted us to pick up the entire cache when cleaning the room rather than having to move the many individual bottles. The dresser also held a small glass container in which we placed pens and pencils to make chart entries. The more convenient your arrangement the smoother your care will be given.

All other supplies for care were kept in the bathroom, which was located only a few feet from Larry's bed. If your bathroom is not close by, you might keep supplies you need frequently in another easy-to-reach place.

The nurse will train the family to properly administer medication and to correctly chart it. You will learn to check the chart often to be sure you are on schedule.

Many drugs have side effects, some patients have an allergic reaction to medication being given, and sometimes interaction of various medications can produce side effects. It is advisable to be aware of the potential for unusual reaction. Doctors or pharmacists will advise you (or you should ask if they don't) of the possible side effects of the prescribed drugs.

Everything taken into the body has an effect upon the whole system. Food, beverages, smoking, vitamins and over the counter nonprescription medications all are processed in the body and change the body chemistry. Sometimes the body is allergic to a food or a food additive. Many people are allergic to milk and milk products. Others cannot eat strawberries or tomatoes because of the acid content. Chocolate is a suspected contributor to migraine headaches. There are those who have bodies that cannot assimilate sugar. They are termed either diabetic or hypoglycemic. Food allergies can be controlled by a proper diet and elimination of foods that cause reactions such as headaches, nausea and discomfort.

If simple food intake can cause disorders in the body, it is important to remember that any medication, whether it be prescription or non-prescription, can also cause changes and reactions in the body. Non-prescription drugs may be even more dangerous than prescription ones because the purchaser takes them without the supervision of a doctor. We cannot assume that just because a drug is sold over the counter without a prescription that it is safe. We must always be aware that *anything* taken into the body can cause a harmful reaction. For instance, if a patient has a cold, do not purchase over the counter, non-prescription drugs to be taken in addition to other medication. Always consult a physician. Let the physician judge the proper cold medication. The nurse or family should also advise the doctor immediately if the patient shows any signs of adverse reaction. Some possible side effects are: nausea, rash, drowsiness, hyperactivity, itchiness, headache, irritability, etc.

Modern medicine has a larger number of drugs now available for the treatment of illness than at any time before in the history of mankind. With this profusion of drugs also comes the heightened danger of side effects. And there is no way of predicting how an individual will react to any drug. Each person has a unique chemical balance. Any ingested substance can change this delicate balance. An example of this is penicillin. The discovery of penicillin, heralded as a wonder drug in combating infections, was one of the panacea of modern drugs that was not without an impediment—allergic reactions. It was quickly noted that some patients suffered side effects.

Besides drugs prescribed for physical illness and disease, over a billion prescriptions were written last year for emotional strain or as an adjunct to psychotherapy. These include mild tranquilizers, appetite depressants and mild sedatives. Analgesics (pain killers) are also included in this category. Many of these can become addictive, either physically or emotionally. All are potentially dangerous to the proper functioning of the human body.

Alchohol itself is a drug. Alcohol combined with any tranquilizer or sedative can be lethal. Many deaths are attributed to the combination of alcohol and drugs. Neither the drug itself nor the alcohol alone would have been fatal, but the combination of the two in the body caused death.

Addiction can develop. Betty Ford recently announced that she had been addicted to both tranquilizers prescribed for neurological pain and to alcohol. She admitted herself to a clinic in order to successfully withdraw from both the drug and the alcohol. A counselor for a local alcoholic rehabilitation agency recently told me that this is a common problem. Alcoholics previously came in with a totally alcohol-related addiction. Now a large percentage take both drugs and alcohol.

Another danger lies in taking more than one prescribed drug. Suppose you go to one doctor and are given a prescription for one ailment. While taking that medication you have another problem, and to to another specialist, who in turn prescribes a medication for that ailment. Either prescription taken alone might have no adverse reaction, but the combination of the two might cause a problem. It is very important that you inform each doctor of the medication you are already taking. Then monitor your own reaction and contact the doctor if you notice any unusual change in either your physical body or your emotions.

Some things to remember about taking drugs:

Short-term vs. long-term treatment: If you have a prescription for a drug that is taken for only a short time, for example, for a sore throat, the drug will remain in the body for a few days after you finish taking the dosage. You must be alert to intake of food and especially alcohol during the entire period the drug is in your system.

If you are taking a prescription for a long-term problem, your body may react differently after you have taken it for a long period of time than it did when you first began.

Also, check with your doctor before taking any medication that you have had on hand for more than thirty days. Drugs may lose or gain potency and can even change their chemical composition.

Be in touch with your own body: No one, not even a doctor, can predict accurately how you will react to any drug. *You* must be the one to determine whether you are experiencing any unusual symptoms. You can then contact the doctor and discuss how you are feeling. He may discontinue the medication and/or substitute another one.

Be sure drugs are taken exactly as prescribed: There is a big difference between taking one pill every four hours and taking four pills every hour. Follow every instruction given. Some medications have specific instructions (one antibiotic carries the instruction that no milk is to be ingested while taking the medication). If the prescription is to be taken *before* meals do not take it in the middle of the afternoon with an empty stomach because you forgot to take it before lunch. Some prescriptions are to be given every four hours (that means that you will have to lose sleep and set the alarm clock at regular intervals) but proper treatment can only be expected if you follow directions carefully. One doctor told of a patient who took all eight tablets (prescribed as two, four times daily) early in the morning because he found it inconvenient to take them at intervals. Then he complained to the doctor because he had a side effect!

Get accurate instructions: Be sure you understand the directions. Written instructions are better than verbal ones to avoid any misunderstanding. Ask the doctor about any possible side effects of the drug in advance.

Take an inventory of your drug habits: How often and how many non-prescription drugs are you taking? How many headaches do you have and how many pills are you taking for relief? What are you taking to help you get to sleep? How often do you need this help? How many "colds" have you had and purchased an over-the-counter drug to cure the symptoms? Are you taking non-prescription pills to reduce appetite and encourage weight loss? How often do you come home from work and need a couple of drinks to help you relax? Do you feel you deserve to drink on weekends because you worked hard all week? How much coffee do you consume each day?

Pills can temporarily relieve symptoms but are not effective in solving life problems. If you are looking for a magic pill to put your life back together, you may be in for another problem caused by taking drugs. That is the problem of addiction, side effects and possibly death. Only *you* have the information to make this evaluation. Only you can contact a doctor to receive help and only you can change your drug habits. Taking an inventory is the first step.

Never, under any circumstances, take any medication that has been prescribed for someone else. The drug or the dosage may not be right for you.

Do not increase the dosage of a drug without consulting your physician. If one tablet gives mild relief don't assume that two would be better. Take all medication exactly as prescribed and if you are not satisfied with the results and are not getting the relief you want, consult the doctor. He may prescribe something else. He may even increase the dosage. But you need supervision and should not indiscriminately adjust the dosage.

There are several books out now that outline drugs and side effects. You can get these in either your local library or bookstore. Your pharmacist is another good source of accurate information.

Cleanliness

Clean hands are a must for all kinds of home care. Keep a supply of bacteria eliminating soap in your bathroom for cleaning hands. Hands should be washed each time you enter the patient's room, and especially before giving medication. Sterile gloves required for decubitus and catheter care may be purchased in a drug store.

If a patient is physically handicapped or weakened by illness, he will need assistance with bathing. The nurse or the physical therapist will determine the amount of help the patient will need, procedures for safety in the bathing process and any equipment that needs to be installed in the tub and shower area. They will also train the family members to assist patients with bathing.

Depending on the condition of the patient, you can give bed baths, or help him take a shower or tub bath.

Bed Baths

If the person is handicapped or too weak to get out of bed you will need to give a bed bath. Your two objectives are: to get the patient clean and to keep him warm.

You will need two containers: one for soapy water and one for rinse water. If a sink is nearby you can use the sink for the soapy water and keep the rinse water near the bed. If you do not have a bedside table large enough to accommodate all your supplies, you might keep a snack tray handy for this use. Use two wash cloths, one for soap and one for the rinse. Have one towel ready for drying. Lay other towels along one whole side of the patient's body to keep the sheets dry. To avoid chills, keep the lower portion of the body covered while you bathe the upper portion. Then cover the top of the body with either a sheet or a clean towel while you are doing the lower portion. Learn to wash in sections, beginning with the face, neck and upper torso. After you have the entire front of the body cleaned, move clean towels to line the opposite side of the body. Turn your patient onto these clean towels to enable you to do the back of the torso and legs. While the patient is still in this position and the bath is complete, you can change the sheets. Push all soiled sheets against the patient's body, along the entire length of the bed. Tuck clean sheets along the side of the bed or under mattress, smooth out and push clean sheets up against patient's body also. At this point you should have clean linen on about a third of the bed. Turn or roll the person *over both* sets of sheets, onto the clean portion of bed. (On a narrow bed take care the patient does not roll off.) Remove the towels, the soiled sheets and then pull out the clean sheets to make up the bed. The patient can now remain on this side or may be moved onto the back if preferred. Remove top sheet and replace with clean one.

Shampoo

Shampooing may be done at any time but is most convenient when done immediately prior to the bed bath. You can shampoo the hair by using a waterless shampoo. This can be purchased in drugstores or at hospital supply departments. This is not a powdered shampoo, but a liquid which looks and smells like any good wet shampoo. It is poured on the hair, head is lathered and rubbed until foam disappears, and toweled dry. A towel under the head keeps the pillow dry. After shampooing, the towel can be removed and the pillow case changed.

Manicure and Pedicure (if permitted by doctor)

As you bathe the patient you can check nails. It is good to clean under nails after each bath and be sure that the cuticle is clean and healthy. Watch for any sign of redness or ingrown nails which are dangerous sites of infection. Manicures and pedicures can be done as needed, but probably will be done once a month. Do this immediately after bathing while the nails are still moist and soft. Use a large towel under hands and feet to catch clippings and keep the bed clean. Some patients (diabetics, paraplegics, etc.) need professional care. Advise the doctor if you note any sign of redness or infection.

Showers

Showers are comfortable and more desirable than bed baths if the patient is mobile. A bath bench placed in the shower can be used if the patient is not strong enough to stand for long periods of time. The success of assisting with the patient's showers depends on how wet the nurse or family member wants to get.

If family members feel comfortable doing so, they can shower at the same time as the patient. This was a real time saver for me when Larry was well enough to get into the shower. I helped him get scrubbed and while he did what he could for himself, I scrubbed myself. Since there was no way to avoid my getting wet when he showered, I simply used this to my advantage and showered with him. It gave us a chance to do one more thing together, and it did save me a lot of time. I always got out first, dried off very quickly and then helped him out into the wheelchair which was covered with a large towel. He sat in the wheelchair while I finished drying him.

If you cannot get into the shower with the patient, wear a bathing suit and shower cap, or some clothing that you don't mind getting wet. In this case you can change clothes after the patient is comfortably back in bed. If you can get into the shower, you can give more assistance to the patient and you can close the door so the bathroom floor will stay dry. If you do not want to get in with the patient, you will have to leave the door open part way and reach in to assist with the bathing. In this case, you will need to spread towels over the floor in front of the shower to avoid slipping on the wet floor.

After the shower is completed, use this opportunity while the patient rests to clean up the bathroom. Since everything is moist from the steam of the bath, and you have plenty of damp towels, you can quickly wipe up walls, floors, shower door, sink, etc., and this saves housekeeping time.

Since the patient usually rests after either a shower or bed bath, you can do the clean-up of the bathroom, dress yourself, and have a little time to catch up on anything you need to do. Soft background music during this time helps patients relax easily and quite often they will take a short nap.

Tub Baths

Patients with good mobility can take tub baths, but should always be assisted in getting in and out of the tub. A bath bench is also helpful in the tub as well as in the shower to allow patients to sit comfortably so they won't become overly tired. It is also easier for patients to sit down at bench level than it is to sit down in the bottom of the tub.

Regardless of the type of baths patients have, the nurse and family members can use the bathing routine to check the patient's general body condition. Patients sometimes become sensitive about having their entire body checked each day. Bath time provides a perfect opportunity for the nurse and family to unobtrusively examine all areas of the body. Some things to check are: general skin condition (dryness, redness, decubitus ulcers), thick, puffy areas on hands, legs, feet, (edema—indicating body tissue is retaining fluid), swelling in any area of the body, rash, moles or warts for unusual appearance, and signs of infections.

Once when I was giving Larry a bed bath, I noticed a lump on his left upper thigh. I carefully noted it and when Lyn came the next day I told her of my discovery. The lump was a beginning abscess and the early discovery allowed us to treat it immediately.

Baths should be given routinely once each day. The time of day can be scheduled to accommodate the patient's wishes and to fit in with other planned events.

A bath and clean linens on the bed can lift a patient's spirits and can become a pleasurable part of their treatment. Patient cleanliness and comfort promote general well-being.

Showers and tub baths can be considered a part of the therapy program. Though they still need assistance with bathing they are getting needed exercise and the immediate goal is to allow them to do as much for themselves as they safely can. The long-range goal is that they will be rehabilitated to the point that they will be able to perform these functions on their own.

Prevention of Bedsores

Bedridden patients or patients who sit in wheelchairs for long periods of time can develop decubitus ulcers—breaks in the skin commonly known as bedsores. An excellent innovative method of preventing this condition is the alternating pressure mattress which consists of many small air pillows. Operating on a small motor which stands at the end of the bed, air is pumped into alternate air pockets every few minutes thus alleviating continuous pressure on any part of the body. As with other patient care equipment, they can be purchased or sometimes are available for loan.

Water beds also help keep the skin in good condition as the water does not apply as much pressure to the skin as a normal mattress. We used a king-sized water bed for Larry not only to protect his skin but to relieve pressure on the spinal cord after he had two laminectomies. Water beds are also helpful if the skin is already broken, decreasing the pressure on the area and giving the skin a chance to heal. If you do not have a water bed and do not want to buy one, water mattresses may be purchased to fit on the top of your regular bed.

It is important to turn patients every two hours to avoid excessive pressure on skin. Patients who are paralyzed, comatose or bedridden for long periods of time need constant skin care. The turning or positioning of patients is also necessary to avoid stiffness developing (contractures, tightening of muscle or tissue around a joint which prevents full motion). The physical therapist can advise the nurse or family of proper positioning techniques.

Healing is promoted by keeping the patient off the tender area as much as possible, allowing for more air circulation and relieving constant pressure which restricts blood flow and slows healing.

One method of healing decubitus ulcers is by drying out the area by applying Maalox, which can be purchased over the counter in any drug store, with a sterile gauze pad. Do not use cotton balls as they stick to the wound and leave fibers. Be careful to *dab gently* and not rub the sentitive tissue of newly forming skin. You can easily scrub away healing tissue. A light is then used to warm the area where the Maalox has been applied. This light can be any goose-necked lamp, using a 75-watt regular light bulb. *Be sure the lamp is at least two feet from the skin and check often* to be sure the skin is drying but not too hot. You want the Maalox to dry but do not want the tender skin to become burned. The light should be used for twenty minutes three to four times per day. Eventually new skin will form if the area is kept dry. Sterile gloves should be used when applying the Maalox and clean pads should be put under the area each time the patient is turned onto the wounded area. Every precaution should be taken to prevent infection. This process should be checked out with the doctor and/or nurse to be sure you are doing it correctly. If you follow the exact instructions, it will work! I learned the procedure in the hospital, and continued the treatment later at home.

Decubitus care must be done with sterile gloves. These open wounds infect easily and every precaution must be taken to avoid infection. If the skin heals over with an underlying infection the wound will have to be reopened for drainage and the whole process of healing will have to be repeated. Occasionally in paraplegic patients the wounds become so severe only surgery will repair the damage.

Bladder and Bowel Care

Proper elimination of waste materials is essential to health. Illness can cause a disruption in a patient's normal bladder and bowel elimination. The nurse and family must routinely assess functioning and adjust diet, fluid intake, exercise and give medication for relief if necessary.

Bladder

Generally, urination is directly affected by fluid intake. To increase the amount of urine, increase the fluid intake. In some cases, the doctor may ask you to measure the amount of fluid intake and output. The nurse supervises this procedure. With specific medical diagnosis, the doctor may determine fluid intake.

Any change from normal such as: dark color or no color at all, large fluid intake and low output, lack of control in voiding, burning, itching or pain, are warning signs. The nurse can evaluate and consult with the doctor for advice.

When patients cannot control the urinary function on their own (called incontinence) due to coma, illness, stroke, paralysis or injury, an indwelling catheter may be inserted into the bladder to ensure flow of urine. Catheters, although providing a support function, can create other complications such as loss of tone of bladder muscle and normal urge to urinate, and recurrent infections. There are alternatives to indwelling catheters which encourage normal function and avoid infections which are difficult to eliminate. Consider those other methods before deciding on an indwelling catheter. External sheath-type for men (also known as Texas catheters) has a condom which attaches to the outside of the penis but has the same hose and bag arrangement for urine collection, if you need to check urine output. It also allows normal functioning of urinary muscles. If the patient is unaware of the passing urine, the placement of a urinal may decrease the incidence of wet bed clothing.

At home, you have the opportunity to try other methods—some of them requiring more effort in care—but the rewards of normal, infection-free elimination are worth any extra effort.

Indwelling catheters require scrupulous hygiene and the procedure for care is critical. The doctor will instruct and order care including irrigation and will set a time for catheter change. Catheters may become blocked and only a professional can make the change safely. A professional may train you to change a catheter, if necessary.

Persistent urinary problems may require a consultation with a urologist or rehabilitation medical staff person, who has had experience with incontinence. Some patients in the spinal cord disability department where Larry was a patient were taught methods to stimulate urination and to do daily catherization when necessary and other methods failed. The primary goal is to restore normal function if possible.

Bowel Care

Normal bowel elimination varies with healthy individuals. It is not necessary to eliminate every day, contrary to television commercials huckstering laxatives. The physical process has become entangled with social and psychological factors. "You cannot possibly be happy if you do not eliminate daily," we are told. The truth is that the relationship between constipation and feeling well has been obscured by commercialism. Patients need to rely on their own pattern of regulation. If constipation does occur and normal rhythm is disrupted, a change of diet, fluid, activity and a relaxed attitude may help. Laxatives should be used only if all else fails. Enemas can empty the lower bowel quickly when needed but can interfere with the normal system and function of the bowel.

Changes such as: color of stool, consistency, blood in stool, pain, burning and itching should be charted and discussed with the nurse or doctor.

The opposite of constipation is diarrhea, a liquid stool, which may be difficult for the patient to control. You need to discover the cause, while treating the diarrhea itself. Continued diarrhea can cause dehydration. Additional fluids should be given during the time the patient has diarrhea.

Constipation and diarrhea are symptoms of temporary imbalance in bowel function, that may be signalling a more serious problem. The condition may be temporary and respond to treatment but a physician should be consulted if the situation persists.

Diet

Getting patients to eat well is most important and often difficult. Illness has a way of destroying appetites, yet the body must have proper nourishment. Life cannot be sustained without food. Vitamin and mineral supplements may be added to the diet but cannot replace the food.

Home care provides the best opportunity for getting a reluctant patient to eat. You can prepare the foods he likes the way he likes them as no hospital can; you can serve his meals when he is hungry and wants them; you can make his mealtime pleasant, his tray attractive. Foods can be served attractively in several rooms of the house and outside in warm weather.

The way food is served is important. The finicky eater may be intrigued by colorful place mats and napkins, pretty dishes, and attractively arranged food.

An everyday diet should include a variety of foods and drinks to provide elements the body needs to be healthy. Doctors may order special diets for patients with certain diseases, which you should carefully follow. A diabetic patient may have a limited sugar diet or a low salt diet may be ordered for patients with heart disease, edema or high blood pressure. Even with restricted diets, there are choices of food and drink. Follow doctor's orders but allow for an occasional treat if some circumstance warrants.

For example, my grandmother is on both a low-sugar and salt-free diet. Her body chemistry gets out of balance if she consumes a larger amount of sugar or salt over a long period of time. She has been on her diet for several years and her weight, her edema and diabetes are well regulated by her diet. If a special event occurs, such as her birthday, we serve her a piece of cake. It would be cruel to be rigid in her diet at this point in her life. She is ninety years old. She enjoys family celebrations very much, especially her own birthday. We would not, of course, deviate from her diet regularly.

People who are ill, whether in the hospital or at home, can be repulsed by large portions of food. It is better if they eat what is served and request more food if they are still hungry. If the person is accustomed to eating "three square meals a day," serve small portions of a variety of foods. It is even more advisable to serve light quantities at short intervals. For instance, instead of serving fruit with lunch, give it in mid-afternoon. Patients who are not getting normal exercise to burn off calories should not overeat. They may develop a weight problem or have difficulty with elimination.

Mealtime should be pleasurable. Patients enjoy having company at mealtime and a waning appetite may be stimulated by your sitting down to eat with them or invite others in to share mealtime. This is an added opportunity to share time together.

Besides providing nutrition, the diet can be used to assist total treatment. If a patient is constipated, you can add more roughage to the diet to stimulate proper elimination. If the problem continues the doctor may need to order a stool softener. There are foods which will help to decrease loose stool also. Your physician may encourage a special diet for this condition.

If a patient has difficulty with solid foods, a soft diet can be planned. Sometimes extremely ill patients cannot even tolerate a soft food diet. You can still provide an appetizing variety of nourishing food in liquid form. Use a blender to make drinks that patients can tolerate. As a base you can use any kind of juice, milk, broth or water. Fresh fruit, sherbet, ice cream, yogurt, wheat germ, protein powder, eggs, and fresh vegetables can be added to make a number of recipes. Blenders can also liquify foods. Stew can be made into a hearty, thick soup that is nutritious and easy to digest. If you are concerned about fluid intake, these drinks will increase the amount of liquid and produce a variety of nutrients.

Even with your best efforts in promoting a nutritious program you may find your patient is not getting the vitamins and minerals needed for maintaining his body. Blood tests may indicate a lack of some mineral and the doctor will prescribe supplements. You can also advise the doctor if you feel your patient is not getting sufficient food intake.

You may also want to study further into the use of nutrition in the healing process and there are a number of books out on the subject.

Dr. Paavo O. Airola, Ph.D., N.D., has written *How To Get Well,* a complete description of all vitamins and minerals, what they do for the body, and what foods provide them. Another book on nutrition, food, vitamins, minerals, diseases, the natural healing process, and an explanation of theories and practical applications of healing techniques is *The Practical Encyclopedia of Natural Healing* by Mary Bricklin.

These books would not replace professional treatment but may help you become more knowledgeable about your body and its functions, option for natural care, the importance of proper food intake, and the use of vitamin and mineral supplements.

MORE THAN JUST THE CARE OF THE PHYSICAL BODY

"A patient is not a machine with a broken part," said Dr. Howard Posner, former chief of the infectious disease division at Lincoln Hospital in New York City and assistant professor of internal medicine at Albert Einstein Medical School, also in New York. Dr. Posner was interviewed by Bill Gottlieb for an article which appeared in the June, 1978 issue of *Prevention* Magazine (pages 74-78). Dr. Posner recently resigned his job to pursue alternative and natural healing methods in his private practice.

"A doctor must have health to give health," Dr. Posner is quoted as saying. "And health for Dr. Posner means health for the whole person: spirit, mind and body—and family. The patient and his family are a unit. I deal with an illness not as an individual problem but as a family problem, as a reflection of what goes on in the family."

I know very little about automobile maintenance. When I had a problem with a noisy muffler I took my car to a muffler specialist who quickly and expertly replaced the tail pipe. When I mentioned to the mechanic that my door wouldn't close tight, he told me, quite politely, that he did not fix doors! Fortunately, I have a good mechanic who looks after my whole car. He fixed the car door, did a routine lubrication and oil change and did a preventive maintenance check.

"The next time you bring the car in we should do a complete tune-up, so plan to leave it with me at least a day," the mechanic told me. I've know this mechanic for over twenty years. He has serviced my cars for that entire time. When he tells me to bring it in for a tune-up, I plan to do exactly what he says because he knows my car and he is a professional.

If it is important to have someone to look at your total car—how much more important it is to have a doctor who can evaluate your whole person. It is sometimes to your advantage to see a specialist for the best results for one particular ailment. But it is also important to have one doctor to look at you as a whole person.

Many doctors are beginning to recognize that the flow of patients in and out of their offices reveals more of a problem than physical symptoms alone. The country doctor who knew all of his patients and who made house calls was well aware of the background lives and situations which affected the disease.

In an article entitled, "Helping Doctors Understand the Patient As Well As the Disease," (*San Francisco Chronicle,* December 24, 1978) writer Richard Saltus talks about: "a novel course at the University of California Medical Center aimed at curing a modern problem: the unfeeling M.D. At a time when medical schools are criticized in some quarters for turning out skilled but unfeeling technicians, U.C. Medical Center with the help of a grant from the Kaiser

Family Foundation is aiming to restore what it calls the *art* of medicine . . . In the modern medical center, doctors treat a stream of strangers from a range of backgrounds and ethnic groups and have to make an effort to understand their origins.''

Other doctors are becoming aware of the emotional and mental contributions to disease. As the medical profession becomes "holistic," many articles written by doctors are appearing in magazines and newspapers as well as in medical journals. Doctors are writing entire books on the effect of the mind on disease. Dr. Kenneth Pelletier explains the new medicine in *Mind as Healer, Mind as Slayer.*

"Holistic medicine recognizes the inextricable interaction between the person and the psychosocial environment. Mind and body functions as in integrated unit, and health exists when they are in harmony, while illness results when stress and conflict disrupt this process."

Doctors disagree on how much effect emotions have on illness. You can get varying opinions ranging from the body as a totally separate entity, with disease being an intruder into the physical from an outside source (germs, environmental pollution, etc.), to scientists who conclude that all disease is caused by a mind set which disrupts the body's natural defense mechanisms and allows disease to take root in the body. In between these two extremely opposite opinions are many doctors who accept the theory of some correlation of the mind and the body, i.e. that any physical disease can affect a patient's emotional or spiritual state and any emotional or spiritual upset can bring about physiological change. Since the mind and spirit are housed in the physical body it is difficult to define them as separate parts.

Health may then be defined as a balance of mind, body and spirit, and disease (sometimes called dis-ease) as an imbalance.

There is a movement growing in popularity in the health field called "holistic." In reading and checking many holistic practices, however, I have found some of them not to be what I define as "holistic," that is, treating the whole person but specializing in some one facet of treatment. I would caution any reader to carefully check holistic practitioners and if they do not include physical care via scientific medicine, an understanding of the emotional (mental) and spiritual potential—they are not holistic. It may be that you will need three or more doctors to treat your three parts (body, mind and spirit)—but do not be misled into thinking you are getting full care if your doctor only practices one facet of treatment.

As doctors become more aware of the need for a holistic approach, it is also important that you, as a patient, understand your own body and its functioning and your responsibility in maintaining health, preventing disease, and/or treatment of disease. The answer to disease originates with you. Doctors will not come to your door and ask if you need medical care. If you are aware of some symptom that is abnormal for you, you must seek medical, emotional or spiritual help. Patients who are aware of a problem and do not seek help immediately run a risk of further complications and handicap the doctor who did not have the opportunity to deal with the symptom when it was in an initial stage. For instance, if a woman discovers a lump in her breast but neglects to go to a doctor immediately, waits a year and then goes to the doctor for advice, she has eliminated any knowledge of what would have been found had she gone in for diagnosis immediately. She will probably feel anxiety about not having it checked, and expects the doctor to miraculously cure her when, in fact, it was her hesitation in seeking treatment that caused the problem. Do not limit your doctor unnecessarily. He can only serve you when you ask him for help. And the sooner the better.

O. Carl Simonton, M.D., in a book co-authored with his wife, Stephanie Matthews Simonton and James Creighton entitled *Getting Well Again,* makes this statement in the very first line of the book: "Everyone participates in his or her health or illness at all times." Later he says "Understanding how much you can participate in your health or illness is a significant first step for everyone in getting well."

The San Diego psychiatrist, Dr. Harold H. Bloomfield, has written a book about the holistic movement. His tip for preventive holism in many cases is just good simple living habits. He offers his suggestions about health, diet, nutrition, smoking and drinking. His book is entitled *The Holistic Way to Health and Happiness.* A book review in the *San Francisco Chronicle,* September 12, 1978, states, "What is different about the holistic health movement is the degree of emphasis on self-reliance for health—something many more conventional treatment-oriented doctors fail to impress on their patients."

Do not expect the doctor to do for you what only you can do yourself. Mechanics can fix your car, they can replace worn out parts, they can repair smashed fenders, they can do preventive maintenance . . . but they cannot drive the car for you. Doctors cannot live your lives for you; like the mechanic, they can only repair and treat and advise. If the mechanic repairs your car often enough, he might be wise to suggest that you take a course in driver training. And the doctor might advise that you make some changes in your life style if you have repeated medical problems. The mechanic can keep replacing the brake linings if you want, but it would be better if you learned not to misuse the brakes on your car. The doctor can keep treating you for a bleeding ulcer but it might be better if you discovered why you had the bleeding ulcer, and take steps to correct the cause.

Only you can seek help and follow good advice.

Attitude

Your orientation to life—how you view yourself, your family, your friends, your job, the world— has an important bearing upon how you will react to an illness or injury. If you are high-strung, tense, negatively based, overly serious, have a tendency to complain, feel you get all the bad luck, or expect the worst, you will carry your thoughts and feelings into a trauma situation.

If, on the other hand, your basic orientation to life is relaxed, calm, essentially positive, you have a tendency to see some good in everything, feel you get your share of good breaks in life, have a sense of humor, and expect the best in every situation—you, too, will carry those feelings into any medical situation. Doctors with whom I have talked agree that patients with a good mental and emotional attitude do better medically. Even with the most serious problems the quality of life can be better.

Does that mean that if you feel angry you should walk around smiling at everyone? Certainly not! It is far better to safely and creatively express the anger, understand why you are angry and work out some solution to the situation. I'm speaking of your basic orientation to life. I am referring to your basic personality. And the way you react to outer circumstances. If you do not handle the little, minor problems well—the chances are greater that you will not react well to larger problems.

Attitudes are thoughts formed in the mind, and attitudes, like every other thought process, can be changed. People are not static, they have potential for change. It is to your advantage to change those attitudes which limit healing, make you ill, and cause you to be unhappy. Events do not make you unhappy—but how you *feel* about the event or what you *think* about the event can make you unhappy. You can live your life as a reactor—letting circumstances control the outcome of a situation or you can act on the circumstances by changing your attitude. For instance: if you lose a leg, you can give up, consider yourself a hopeless invalid, center your thinking on the leg you've lost, and limit your life in all areas of relationships. Or you can be grateful that you're alive, center your thinking on the talents and abilities you have, consider yourself a whole person and live a full life.

In both cases you will have lost a leg, but the quality of life you have will depend entirely on your attitude.

Larry and I had a friend who had a heart attack about fifteen years ago. He was a veterinarian in a small mid-west city. He wrote us that the heart attack was a marvelous experience. During his recuperation he had the time to examine his life. He said it changed his priorities and because of the seriousness of his illness, he felt grateful to be alive. He mentioned thinking of all the worries he thought he had and how insignificant they were, compared to life itself.

Our body sends us messages when we are ill. If we've mis-used it, pushed it past its limits, refused to stop our activities when the body signaled "tired," or neglected it in any way—illness can be a flashing red light to gain our attention. We may be able to assist in our own healing—we may have to live with a body that's sick. In either case, our attitude will determine the kind of life we will have.

Humor As Healer

Eric Berne, M.D., in his book *Games People Play,* states: "Hopefulness, enthusiasm or a lively interest in one's surroundings is the opposite of depression; laughter is the opposite of despair."

The story of Norman Cousins' illness and amazing recovery has two factors with which I totally agree. Norman Cousins described his experience in an article in the *Saturday Review* on May 28, 1977. It has also recently been told in his book, *Anatomy of an Illness as Perceived by the Patient: Reflections on Healing and Regeneration.* His description parallels many theories now being explored about the cause of illness being the effect of negative emotions on the human body and the reversal of those symptoms when the mental attitude of the patient changes. This change in attitude brings into focus a strong will to live.

After receiving a diagnosis of ankylosingspondylitis in 1954, which the doctors considered incurable, Cousins began his own unconventional treatment. The first part was a change in attitude. To help this process he prescribed for himself large doses of laughter to stimulate a positive attitude. He picked comedy television programs to watch daily. His second decision for self-treatment was to take large intravenous doses of Vitamin C. There is controversy in cases like Norman Cousins, where patients get well despite the hopeless medical diagnosis. Whether or not you believe in Vitamin C as a body healer or whether you believe that attitude plays any part in either causing the physical illness or in the recovery process—I hope you will believe in the power of the patient in making his own decision about his life, his illness, and how he wants to live out whatever days he has to live in his own way.

Norman Cousins describes a recent chance meeting with one of the doctors who made the terminal diagnosis of his illness. The doctor was obviously puzzled and surprised at Cousins' apparent health and vitality. Cousins' comment was that he hoped doctors would be more careful about making "pronouncements of doom." The danger, he stated, was that patients would believe the experts and "that would be the beginning of the end."

Dr. Raymond A. Moody, Jr., author of *Life After Life* has written a new book entitled *Laugh After Laugh—The Healing Power of Humor.* In it he states: "As a society we appear to have become obsessed with the notion that there ought to be a pill or an operation or a machine to treat each illness. We tend to think that the doctor should be able to cure us—instantaneously, preferably—of any ailment, with a minimum of effort or cooperation on our own part. Such magical attitudes about the efficacy of modern technological medicine have led to a neglect of the very factors of emotion and mental outlook which may precipitate disease, and affect its course, duration and outcome. Hopefully, focusing for awhile on the relationship between humor and health may help to correct this imbalance, at least to some degree."

Dr. Moody writes about the history of humor and medicine, citing examples of healing and explains how humor works in healing.

Sometimes people asked me how Larry and I could stand living with a "terminal" illness—that it must have been very depressing. I always found this question puzzling because our lives were exciting and fun before the illness and exciting and fun (albeit in a different way) after the cancer diagnosis. Larry and I found humor in many situations.

Once when Larry was in the hospital and had not had a good appetite, he surprisingly announced one winter's evening that he had a craving for watermelon. A friend of Larry's set out to find a watermelon, hampered by the fact that it was nearly closing time for the local markets and that watermelons were out of season. About an hour later our friend appeared at the door with a large, whole watermelon which he ceremoniously placed on Larry's bedside tray table.

"Well, all we need now is a sharp knife," I said.

Larry looked up and said with all seriousness—"Maybe we can take it to the operating room to get it cut up."

Fortunately our friendly nurse arrived to take his temperature. "Where did you get the big watermelon?" she asked.

She and I teased Larry because the only times we'd crave watermelon in winter was when we were pregnant. She asked Larry if he was sure the doctor's diagnosis was correct.

While Larry sat in bed with the thermometer in his mouth, the nurse disappeared. When she returned, she had a steak knife, four plastic forks and four plastic cups with removable plastic liners. We "plugged" the watermelon, making sure we only cut it on the top to avoid a mess. Then we all ate cubes of what everyone agreed was the best watermelon we had ever tasted. Not only did the watermelon help Larry's eating problem, and provide a comic relief to a serious situation, it provided an opportunity for the nurse, the patient and the family to relate in a healthy way.

Books, comics and cartoons, television and movie comedies all bring laughter out of otherwise serious and tragic subjects. The humor is there if we will only see and enjoy it.

William Fry, psychiatrist, and Melanie Allen, Ph.D., filmwriter and psychologist, co-authored a book on humor entitled *Make 'Em Laugh,* in which they discuss the relationship between humor and creativity, particularly as it applies to television and movie comedy writers. The authors interviewed seven successful writers, who described their motivations for writing comedy, their philosophies and benefits of laughter to mankind. The authors describe humor as, "everyone's everyday magic." They also state, "To the humanistic psychologist, humor is a means of actualizing one's self while coping with life's ups and downs."

The comedy writers felt that not only did they feel they were contributing to the world but that their own lives were improved by humor. In fact, they began careers in writing humor because they found the benefits in their own lives and developed a knack of seeing the whole of life through the eyes of humor.

There is a tie between the opposites of tragedy and humor. In the fourth century B.C. the Greek Theatre presented two kinds of plays, tragedy and comedy. They wore masks in these plays to denote the type—one a tragic face, the other a smiling face. These masks of comedy and tragedy have become the symbols of drama and have survived the centuries that have passed. But the masks are not separated, as life is not separated. The masks are overlapping, and events in life are both tragic and comic at the same time. Humor eases the pain of tragedy and tragedy balances out comedy. Comedy merely exaggerates tragic circumstances.

On Halloween I had an appointment to visit a hospital chaplain. As I waited, a group of high school students arrived. Some were dressed like clowns in colorful costumes. All wore masks or had heavy makeup and wigs. I noticed the reaction of the people in the waiting room. Everyone—the hospital receptionist, passing medical staff and worried family members, responded to their presence. As the teenagers sang and laughed, the atmosphere in the waiting room changed. They had come to visit the children in the pediatric ward but they brightened the lives of everyone they met. If Dr. Moody is right—and humor is healing—maybe the world needs more clowns.

Leisure, Recreation, Hobbies, Social Life

Leisure time in home care is essential to balance out structured nursing care (bathing, dressing, taking medication and eating). Even though these nursing chores can be done at the patient's own pace, they are a reminder that the patient is ill. Leisure time provides a freedom from routine care and gives the patient a chance to relax and use the time in any constructive way he chooses. Primarily I consider leisure to be quieting, or passive. Even sleep is a good use of leisure time provided it is not overdone. If you find your patient is using leisure time to retreat into sleep (a good escape from the reality of illness) as opposed to a restful nap, you may need to suggest more recreational activities.

Recreation (re-creation) involves any activities that are interesting to the patient. Recreation can include hobbies and social events, but can also include any activity in which the patient actively participates. The more ambulatory the patient, the wider choice of activities you have. Car trips, even for a short duration, offer a welcome change of scene, a variety of places to visit, and the chance to fill deprived senses with sights of the outdoors.

Sometimes Larry would accompany me on routine shopping trips. I didn't find them especially stimulating but Larry found them exciting. If a patient cannot get out in the car, get him out into the yard or patio, if possible. Rather than leave Larry in the house when I had gardening to do, I'd wheel him outside onto the patio while I weeded or watered. He sometimes took wild bird seed to attract and feed the birds, or he'd sit and watch the humming bird feeder, "waiting for a customer," he said. We sometimes read or had lunch together on the patio. Simple things become a pleasant recreation when done outdoors.

If you have a patient who is bedridden or confined to the house you will need to use other ways to provide diversion and stimulate the senses. Lyn brought some special record albums which she played while doing the bathing or other nursing chores. One was a record of southern music: Stephen Foster medleys, "Dixie," and "Shenandoah," which was one of Larry's favorites.

Music is a great emotional elevator or calmer, geared to patients' preferences. It can also be used to reverse patients' moods. If they are discouraged some jazz or "beat" music can lift the mood. If they are trying to rest or relax, soft, soothing music can assist the relaxation.

The television, radio and phonograph all offer entertainment for the patient. Used alternately to afford variety, they have greater value. Too much TV viewing or too much time spent listening to the radio tends to make the patient overly passive. The object is to use them in conjunction with other more strenuous activities. The TV set should never become a pacifier or replacement for warm human relationships. A favorite TV program after dinner can provide a diversion while the family washes the dishes and cleans up the kitchen. All of these media inventions provide a marvelous link to the outside world and help patients keep a perspective of life as it exists for other people. It is always good therapy when you can broaden their focus.

Patients who are not mobile enough to change channels by operating the set themselves can be provided with a remote control switch. A small, portable radio kept either on or near the bed that they can control is better than a large expensive model that requires assistance to operate. The more they can do for themselves, the more decisions they can make unaided—no matter how small—the more independent they will feel. No one likes to be totally dependent upon another person. Somehow self-worth gets mistakenly aligned with being self-sufficient. Self-worth, of course, really has nothing to do with your ability to function—or your performance. But many patients do equate the two.

When Larry spent most of the time in bed, we introduced two new hobbies: coin and stamp collecting. Larry and Lyn read books on the history of coins and stamps, what makes them valuable, and tips on collecting. Some friends visited with their fourteen-year-old son who brought along his stamp collection. He was quite knowledgeable about stamps and he and Larry spent most of the visit looking at and talking about stamps.

Each night when I came home Larry asked me to empty all of my change on his desk-tray and he would look over the coins to see if they were valuable. We bought a few coins and stamps which Larry carefully selected. If he had a question, he'd pick up the telephone and call either a coin or stamp store owner. His interest grew and these became active new hobbies for him.

Larry had been an avid reader all his life. It was only natural that he would take advantage of the time recuperation provided to do reading he would not have been able to do had he been well. I went to the library and either got books that he requested or would select some books myself. One day as I was returning some overdue books, I explained to the woman working at the desk that the books were late because I found it difficult to get all my errands done after work while caring for my husband at home. She introduced me to Friends of the Library and the services they provided: bringing books to the home, visiting with patients to learn of their interests, and providing a pickup and delivery service. It was another opportunity to have someone from the community come in for a visit and it relieved me of one task.

I found not only were books available, but books recorded on tape cassettes and records for those who could not read. This service is available nationwide. If you are interested, contact the library in the area where you live.

Photography was another of Larry's long-time interests. After he had had cancer for more than two years, he decided to take a correspondence course in photography. It took more than two years to complete but he was so proud when he received his certificate of completion and a card on which was printed, "Free-Lance Photographer." Although he had always enjoyed photography, he developed an interest into a professional hobby only after he became ill.

Completing the photography assignments became another thing we could do together. One of his first assignments was to photograph a community building and in some way identify the building's use in the photograph. At the time the photography assignment was due, Larry made one of his unexpected trips to the hospital. During his recuperation period after surgery he asked me to bring the camera so he could complete the assignment on time. He took some shots of the side of the hospital building showing the emergency room entrance, which clearly showed the use of the building as required in the assignment. In order to get the proper camera angle I had to wheel Larry into the parking area. You can imagine what a surprise our outing was to Larry's surgeon who drove by in his car.

This was not the first time Larry took photographs at a hospital. Larry had looked forward to the arrival of our first grandchild. He sat in his wheelchair at the end of the corridor while our daughter, Carol, was in the labor room. Together, we heard Nicky's first cry. The nurse wheeled Nicky in a glass-enclosed bassinet past the doorway on the way to the nursery, and we saw our grandson, wide-eyed and alert, for the first time.

The next day we returned and joined the ranks of new grandparents who lined up to get their first views of the new arrivals. I looked at the name tags. My eyes found the correct basket. I looked at the baby, sound asleep on his side, facing the window glass. "Larry!" I exclaimed. "Look at the red hair!"

"His mother is blonde, his father's hair is brown," I felt compelled to explain to the grandmother standing next to me whom I had startled with my outburst.

"His hair *is* red," Larry answered. "I always wanted red hair," I said. "My grandfather, several great aunts and cousins had red hair. Some of the relatives thought I might have children with red hair but I never in my wildest dreams ever thought about my grandson having red hair." Of course we thought he was beautiful. Larry took many pictures of Nicky through the nursery glass enclosure.

Larry did well during Nicky's first months of life. Sometimes Larry drove down to Carol's home and took her and Nicky to lunch. Sometimes he'd just stop in to take pictures of Nicky sitting in his high chair or swing. All of the pictures he recorded for our family album were exceptional.

Larry usually used a 35mm camera but he also purchased a camera that developed prints immediately which he used to photograph visitors so he could give them the prints.

One of the greatest benefits of home care is the opportunity to provide a full social life for the family. We geared invitations according to how Larry was feeling. When he felt good, we would plan more organized events. When he was not feeling well, we simply let people drop in to visit for as long as he wanted. Even on days when he did not feel like long visits, he at least had the emotional support of knowing that someone cared enough to stop by to see him.

Larry liked all kinds of activities. Sometimes we would invite another couple for dinner on weekends when I was off from work and could make preparations. This took some organization and planning but was always worth the effort. I would usually plan an "oven dinner," which required little last minute preparation. Combined with either a gelatin or tossed green salad (which could be prepared in advance and stored in the refrigerator) and a dessert which I purchased at a nearby bakery, I could turn out attractive and tasty meals with a minimum of work. Since Larry was on an unrestricted diet, I had a wide choice of entrees. Oven meals included pot roast of beef surrounded with vegetables, swiss steak, chicken, any number of ways, and occasionally spare ribs, a favorite of Larry's. Main dish casseroles with meat and cheese were also easy to prepare in advance. Vegetable casseroles could be used as side dishes to the main course.

The dinners called for careful organization. I prepared all food possible early in the day. Most nursing chores were completed by mid-afternoon, including bathing Larry and changing bed linen. Late in the afternoon, while Larry either napped or rested, I bathed, put on make-up and dressed for the evening, after which all food went into the oven, timing everything so that the meal would be ready at the time I wanted to serve. The table was set in advance, with colorful flowers or place mats to make the dinner more festive.

Larry usually remained in bed to conserve his energy until the guests arrived. After I greeted our visitors and got them comfortably settled in the living room, I served them some snack food and drinks. Then I helped Larry into his wheelchair and we joined the guests. From that point on, we could have been any couple entertaining. Larry's wheelchair pushed under the dining room table easily and we enjoyed sharing meals in the dining room with friends. After dinner we sat in the living room by the fireplace in cold weather or on the patio in warm weather and continued our conversation begun over dinner. Occasionally we played cards or dominoes but Larry enjoyed the opportunity to converse more than he liked playing games. When the guests were ready to leave, Larry and I escorted them outside. It was not as attractive to take them through the garage to the street, but Larry's wheelchair ramp was installed from the main hall through the garage into the front driveway. It was more important for Larry to be able to escort his guests out than to have them leave by the more attractive main entrance, and none of our guests complained.

I immediately helped Larry back into bed, where he could rest while I did last minute clean-up. Later, when I rejoined him in the bedroom, we would talk about the night's events while I gave him his medication, finished making entries on the daily chart, and helped him prepare for sleep.

During the week we sometimes invited people over for coffee and dessert. We could still have our social time together but the planning was much simpler than doing a full dinner.

Sometimes Larry did not feel well enough to get up in his wheelchair when we had guests, like the time we celebrated Nicky's first birthday. Larry had helped select Nicky's gifts and I ordered a birthday cake. Lyn cooked a large "pot" of food since I worked that day and we ate "family style." When dinner was served, Larry wanted to eat dinner in his room, so Steve took a tray and joined him. When it came time for Nicky to open his gifts, we all gathered in Larry's room so he could participate in the party and share the happiness of this first birthday celebration.

The only activities not carried out in Larry's room were the messy process of having Nicky eat his first piece of birthday cake and when Nicky wanted to play with some of the noisy toys he received as gifts. Noises sometimes made Larry tense, which contributed to his pain.

Larry took many birthday pictures from his bed. We were careful to watch Nicky closely so that his ever-increasing curiosity did not place Larry in any danger. With proper awareness, visits were fun and Larry enjoyed watching Nicky's growth. During babies' first years they change quickly and Larry watched new abilities develop.

Our son, John, came in and out at various times of the day. His job required split-shift work. His arrival was always a happy time for Larry. John would walk into the room saying, "Hi, Dad, how goes it?" Larry would smile and John would continue walking around the bed and lean over to give Larry a hug. Then he'd pull up a chair and they'd spend a few minutes talking about the day's activities.

John and Larry both had a sense of humor and I could hear their laughter echoing in other parts of the house. John's return home and being with Larry freed me to do work in another part of the house.

In a long-term situation, it is not wise to allow the patient to become dictatorial, demanding house rules that allow no freedom for other family members. Nor is it fair to have family members setting life patterns that do not take into consideration the patient's illness and its demands. Living on the razor's edge is never easy and it is more of an art than a science.

Some conflicts are bound to occur in daily living. Having an ill member of the family can only add to the frequency of the conflicts.

There was the time that John decided to sand his car and prepare it for painting. He figured to do the work on his time off from work and by putting in long days at it, he'd soon have it done.

The sound of the sander was heard throughout the house. It buzzed from morning till noon when John broke for lunch, then it was on again. Larry's tolerance to noise was low, and he finally reached his limit. Lyn played records but it didn't cover the racket. The time had come for mediation and Lyn volunteered to hear the discussion when Larry summoned John to the bedroom. A compromise was worked out that didn't quite please either one of them, but was one both could live with.

Just as the patient needs the support of the family, he also contributes to the family. Each member has his own unique contribution to make. When the unit is broken by a hospital confinement, all members feel that absence. Larry said he felt the extreme isolation in the hospital, as if life were continuing for everyone else and he was left on the sidelines.

At home, he could experience everything. He shared in the news of John's promotion on the job, worried about Nicky when he was ill and had a temperature of 104°, helped with arrangements for holidays and special events, and cried when he read that Martha Mitchell, stricken with cancer, had died alone in a hospital room.

Life with all its panorama of emotions was open to him and at home he was a part of it—not just a spectator on the sidelines, but a participant. We all learned and received as much from him as we gave. The family unit was not complete without him. Just his being at home, his help in choosing an appropriate gift, his laughter, his special prayers and comments—his presence—all were precious to us. Larry's illness, like all of his life, was not his alone, it was ours, too.

The extension telephone was placed on Larry's bed. Larry kept a list of names and phone numbers in a folder along with other papers he used often. When Lyn or I were busy with other duties, Larry often made phone calls to friends. He liked having this independence. He sometimes wrote short notes while he sat propped up in bed, using his tray as a desk. At Christmas time he addressed envelopes for cards and wrote short notes to friends.

When he wanted to write a lengthy letter or do an article, he used a tape recorder. I typed a draft of the tapes, which Larry then read and edited before I typed the final copy.

Sometimes, when the pain was worse, Larry's general good nature turned hostile and he would yell at the person closest at hand. We all understood that this would pass and it was merely a manifestation of his pain. We shared it, even though the feeling of desperation and frustration at not being able to stop the pain entirely hurt us, too. At times like that, we did not joke with him as we usually did. We took the pain seriously and allowed him some peace and quiet and solitude. Usually a short time later, his voice would echo through the house as he called our names. This was our signal that the pain had subsided and he was ready for conversation or some other social exchange.

Patients will give what they can in their own way. The trick is for the medical staff and family to allow them to give and be a functioning, active part of the family unit.

How to Solve Boredom: Stimulate not Manipulate

Stimulation may be needed to open areas of creativity or recreation, but I strongly oppose having relationships deteriorate to the point where families feel obligated to "entertain" the patient constantly.

There is as much need for the recreative power of silence, of relaxation; allowing patients to be quiet and alone as there is a desire to keep them from being bored. Patients have many things done to and for them. Sometimes a nice respite and change of pace is to simply leave them alone for awhile—free of treatment, dispensing of pills and nursing care, which takes up so much of their day. And you must be aware of the individual differences in personality. Some people are more inclined to solitary activities and enjoy being alone. Others tend to be more gregarious and like more people-centered activity. The same person may one day need more time alone, while on other days more activity may be needed. Always be considerate of the person's own needs and adjust the schedule of activities accordingly.

For instance, after a physical therapy session, patients may not feel up to playing games or doing anything strenuous, mentally or physically. This might be a good time to straighten up the bed, make them comfortable and let them relax with some good music to create a peaceful atmosphere. The same advice applies after visitors have left—this is a good time for a quiet change of pace.

If you need some things to do to relieve your patient's boredom— always compatible with his personality—you might consider the following:

cards	there are many kinds of card games. Solitaire is a game the patient can play alone—while gin rummy, etc., can be played by two or more. It may be a good time to learn how to play bridge, for instance.
dominoes chinese checkers chess backgammon	good with visitors and family
oil painting or watercolor	a solitary pastime
photography	can provide mental stimulation and opportunity for social exchange.
printing calligraphy creative writing	a solitary pastime
coin collecting stamp collecting	there is more to these hobbies than just collecting.

scrap books or family albums	what family doesn't have pictures, cards, travel souvenirs, etc., that need organizing and mounting. This not only is a time user, but gives the person a feeling of accomplishment. Slides can be sorted and put into trays.
Japanese paper folding	another activity patients can do alone
reading	offers a wide variety of topics
writing letters	either by their own hand or written by family or nurse.
recording on tape tracing family genealogy	to pursue alone or share
music	can quiet and relax or can be used as stimulation.

Man's Best Friend

There are other family members who often are overlooked but who play an important role in the patient's state of well-being. They are the family pets.

People who are devoted to their pets, and that includes nearly everyone who has a pet, feel a great sense of loss when separated from them. Children and the elderly are especially attached to family pets, some of them identifying more strongly with a pet than with other family members.

It has been observed that among elderly persons hospitalized with serious illnesses, the ones who have pets have a greater incentive to get well. Perhaps the feeling of being needed, generated by having a pet dependent upon them for care, made the difference.

Home care provides the only opportunity for patients to be re-united with pets. Institutional rules prohibit the presence of pets. A few brave souls have tried to overcome this barrier, however.

A nurse told me the story of a man confined to a hospital where she was on duty. He was suffering from cancer and she was sure he would not linger for more than a day or two. One day he took her hand and said, "I could die happy if I could only see my dog one more time."

Fortunately for him, the nurse was a pet owner herself and understood his need. Since the patient was in a private room, one that was located on the first floor with a patio opening onto a nearby street, she decided to arrange for the wife to bring the dog the next day. The man was so happy to have his dog spend a few hours with him. No doubt the dog's lying on the bed would have broken all the rules for cleanliness but the visit made the man happy and content. When the man died a day or two later, any violation of hospital policy seemed insignificant compared to the man's peace of mind and satisfaction. The nurse is to be complimented for her sensitivity to her patient's needs and for her strength in being able to act upon what she knew to be the proper priority—a patient's last request over hospital rules.

Larry and I had a cat and fortunately for us, Lyn liked cats. And because of this, "Robert E. Lee" had a special place in our family. His all grey color gave Larry the idea for his name. Larry sometimes laughingly called him "The Confederate General," or the "General." Whether Lyn liked the cat or had a loving prejudice for his southern name, I do not know. But for whatever reason, Robert E. Lee, a third generation member of our cat family, was not evicted from his favorite sleeping place—at the foot of Larry's bed.

Communication

When a member of the family becomes ill, and more particularly, if he is to be cared for at home, there will be more need than ever for open lines of communication. Even more than a crisis, this long-term situation can test the communication within the family.

If there isn't free flow of honest give-and-take, it may be that some effort should be given to understanding communication and how it can work for you.

Communication is the act of imparting knowledge, sharing feelings and/or thoughts with another person or group of persons. There is individual communication between friends, family, acquaintances and a socialized form of communication between groups of people. There is also communication with one's self. Life cannot be lived without communication.

There are many kinds of communication. There is role playing communication where a person communicates as a role rather than as an individual, i.e. on the job, or in situations which require specific behavior appropriate to the circumstances. That is not to say that we do not bring our personality to the situation but that the situation does not allow full communication of our thoughts and feelings . . . that the behavior is primarily determined by our role.

There are verbal and nonverbal communications. Verbal communication relies on the use of words. This attempt to verbalize is hampered by both the inability of the speakers to properly convey their thoughts or feelings and the misunderstanding of the listeners. Words alone do not convey the honest message—nonverbal messages are sometimes transferred through silence or body movements, especially facial expressions. Sometimes words may carry one message and the body another.

Illness, injury, and the trauma they bring into people's lives can complicate or disrupt the normal communication process. It begins with the doctor-patient consultation. In a previous section I discussed the coparticipant relationship between the doctor and patient. The ideal consultation is when the patients provide adequate and factual information about symptoms and doctors diagnose, explain, advise, and outline options for treatment. Patients then have the necessary information on which to base their decision for treatment.

The communication process can be derailed at any point: the patient may not give the doctor an honest evaluation of symptoms. For instance, if a man goes to a doctor complaining of nervousness, sweating, lack of appetite, a general feeling of tiredness and describes a recent weight gain, these symptoms could indicate a number of diseases. The doctor, however, notices that the patient has a "bloaty" look. During the course of the examination, the doctor asks him how much he drinks. "Only occasionally, Doc," the patient lies. The doctor cannot treat the real problem—that of alcoholism—because the patient did not give correct information. The doctor then may run several tests to determine the problem (all very costly to the patient) and may prescribe medication for the symptoms—while the patient continues to drink. Until the patient can recognize and accept the problem for what it is, the doctor has no chance for successful treatment.

Or in another case, a woman with a history of venereal disease does not tell the obstetrician when she becomes pregnant, thus limiting her doctor's ability to properly care for her. Doctors can best treat patients when they have all the information about the patient's past medical experience and the truth about his present symptoms.

The patient may even hint at the real problem but be unwilling to discuss it out of fear of what will be found. "I'm sure it's nothing, doctor, but I sometimes have a little discomfort after eating." After extensive tests, the patient was diagnosed as having a bleeding ulcer. In this case, the patient did seek treatment, but the diagnostic process could have been shortened considerably had the doctor not had to play hide and seek for information.

Another possible communication barrier is when the doctor deals only with the symptom the patient described, and does not deal with larger issues. For instance, an obese patient comes in for treatment of indigestion problems. The doctor will treat that, but will not tell the patient to lose weight or a patient has ulcers and the doctor treats the ulcers but does not discuss what is happening in the patient's life to make him ill. Or the doctor may be perfectly honest and tell the obese patient to lose weight and the patient "misunderstands" or does not hear that part of the diagnosis—because his basic motivation is enjoyment of food, not losing weight or improving digestion. He just wants the digestive process to work well so that he can eat all he wants. The doctor-patient relationship is crucial when you are ill. It deserves the best that each person can bring to it. Honest communication may not be easy, but it is worth any effort needed to build a trusting assocation.

The communication within families is subject to the same processes—the same potential for trusting and honest experiences together. Healthy relationships are not only desirable but are necessary in order to live life to its fullest.

Communication is often ruled by our thoughts and emotions, which involve us in maneuvers, strategems and games (not to be interpreted as fun). Games can become very serious and have drastic consequences.

A. H. Chapman, M.D., (psychiatrist) has written an easy to read, informative book entitled *Put-offs and Come-ons* in which he explains psychological manipulations. He describes "Whine and Decline," a maneuver—when a wife unconsciously knows how to provoke an argument exactly at the time her husband begins sexual advances, and a strategem "Poor Me" in which a patient says, "I could get well doctor, if only you could do something about my husband."

Eric Berne, M.D. in his widely read *Games People Play* defines games as having an outcome which he calls a "payoff." People wouldn't play games if they didn't get something out of them. What Berne calls transactions are a form of communication. He shows a structural diagram of what he calls "a complete personality," consisting of a: Parent/Adult/Child

"Everyone carries his parents around inside of him. Everyone has an adult and everyone carries a little boy or girl around inside of him," Dr. Berne states. He cautions that "child" should not be thought of as *childish* but rather *childlike.*

Berne says "Actually the child is in many ways the most valuable part of the personality, and can contribute to the individual's life exactly what an actual child can contribute to family life: charm, pleasure and creativity.

"The adult is necessary for survival. It processes data and computes the probabilities which are essential for dealing effectively with the outside world.

"The parent has two main functions: first it enables the individual to act effectively as the parent of actual children . . . and it makes responses automatic, which conserves a great deal of time and energy."

In the doctor-patient relationship according to Dr. David Levenson's chart discussed earlier, the first model had this structure:

doctor   (in the terminology of Dr. Eric Berne, this could be
↓   called the parent)
patient   (and the patient could be called the child)

It would be more advisable for both the doctor and patient to communicate from the adult-adult states, like model #2 in Dr. Levenson's chart.

doctor ◄────► patient

Thomas Harris, M.D., in his book, *I'm O.K.—You're O.K. (A Practical Guide To Transactional Analysis),* affirms that "The individual is responsible for what happens in the future, no matter what has happened in the past." Dr. Harris takes Dr. Berne's structural theory of the parent-adult-child and gives it another interpretation, "I'm O.K—You're O.K."

In the medical situation the patient often feels "Not O.K." and thinks of the rest of the world as "O.K." Actually, everyone carries degrees of "O.K." and "Not O.K." simultaneously. If the patient can feel "O.K." and "Not O.K." and realize that everyone else feels "O.K." and "Not O.K." too, a healthier relationship can be established. Dr. Berne describes a state of consciousness where we can become "game free," a state of autonomy.

Dr. Berne has written another book, *What Do You Say After You Say Hello?* I found this book to be easier to understand than his original book, *Games People Play,* which was written for professionals.

I have included these books as resources because it is important to be aware of the complexity of communication and also the opportunities to understand and adjust patterns which are disruptive and destructive. Life is so brief—no matter how long you live—that to miss any chance for real relationship is a tragic waste.

Do not confuse the normal letting out of appropriate emotions with games. When a woman broke her hip for the third time, the doctor told her: the hip is broken *again* and surgery will be required (*again*). She already knew about the long recuperation period and immobility, he did not need to tell her about that. She began to cry. Crying was a form of communication of feelings.

"Don't cry, mother," the daughter said. "Everything will be alright."

The mother's crying was a release of emotion; frustration at having to go through surgery again, anger at being so clumsy and falling in the first place, fear of pain and the discomfort of surgery, sadness at having her life disrupted. The doctor wisely said, "Let her cry. It's a good, normal, healthy reaction!" If, however, the mother is still moping, depressed and crying three weeks later or three months later and she has not moved naturally from the initial emotion, then you have to find out what is happening in her physical, emotional or spiritual life (the whole person). Her continued crying is no longer natural or healthy.

If a patient who is normally "pretty easy going" after a serious illness became increasingly angry and hostile toward the medical staff and family, it is far better to evaluate the whole situation than to ignore it. Part of the evaluation will be to use your knowledge of games, strategems, and maneuvers. You may see yourself described in one of the games—if so, you are most fortunate—because awareness and recognition of a problem are the first essential steps to finding a solution. In this situation as well as all others involving home care, use the strength of the team. You may need professional help to understand and/or free you from games.

Growth in human beings comes as change. And growth, no matter how painful at the time, brings you into a new dimension of life. Open communication is a valuable part of that growth process.

Chapter VI

Burnout

Any book focused on the care of a long-term or a terminal patient in the home would not be complete without a few words directed to the one on whom most of the responsibility rests—you.

By now you have discovered that home care is work. A lot of work. It is laundry and cooking, nursing and grocery shopping, doing dishes at midnight and trying to keep cheerful when the chips are down.

It is also a heavy emotional burden, a sublimation of grief, a gnawing fear of the future, a worry about finances, all of which you may try to conceal. The events that led up to the home care may have cast some reflections on your spiritual life. How could this have happened to us? you may have asked—more than once.

Are you going to accept what appears to be the only logical solution? Work as hard and as long as possible so that when you do get a chance to go to bed you'll be too tired to think and will sleep from pure exhaustion?

I hope not. Because that road leads you straight and inevitably to "Burn out," literally a bankruptcy of your physical, emotional and spiritual bank account. When you have burned up all your energy, how then are you going to care for your loved one who is ill?

There is a better way. By learning how to conserve your strength and to restore your resources you will be making at least as many deposits as withdrawals in your account. It should be considered as one of your most important duties to your patient.

At this point you are probably saying, wearily and resentfully, "Yes, but. . .

101

"But how can I find time for anything *more* when I am juggling dozens of things simultaneously, frantically trying to keep everything going?"

"But what if I can't afford to hire help?"

There are a lot of "buts," and I used them all before I came to the realization that I had to cut away the deadwood of tasks that could be left undone or delegated to someone else; that it was important to save a little time out for myself so that I could build up my nearly depleted physical, emotional and spiritual energy levels.

Home care's first demand, I learned, is to learn to manage time wisely. That's where I started.

Some suggestions are:

—Set up a list of reasonable priorities. It has been said that the whole secret to getting things done is knowing what to leave undone. You'll have to spend less time on some things and cut out others altogether. You will not be able to do everything. Learn to cut corners—cook double batches of food and freeze one portion for another day—quit trying to be the perfect housekeeper you were before. And *don't* feel guilty about the dust on the piano.

—Organize your work. Become a list-maker. A good way to start is by listing everything that has to be done during the day, in the order of their priority. It relieves you of the stress of carrying all of the details in your mind. You can cut your errand-running and shopping time in half if you organize your lists, separated according to the items you need to buy and places you have to go—bank, filling station, post office, dry cleaners—then arrange a logical itinerary. I suggest you buy only items you have on the list to save money and prevent compulsive shopping, which is a time waster. Saves time and gasoline, too,

—Keep supplies you use often in or near the patient's room. A pitcher of ice water on the bedside table will save you many trips to bathroom or kitchen. A paper sack (I used lunch sacks because they looked more attractive) pinned to the mattress with a safety pin will keep tissues, gum wrappers and other flotsam and jetsam that collects as if by magic, from becoming litter that has to be picked up. A wastebasket for dressings, sterile gloves and the morning newspaper should be kept somewhere near the bed. For the patient who is bed-ridden but active enough to require entertainment, a canvas tote bag for magazines, books, notebook, deck of cards, brush and comb, mirror and cigarets, etc. will keep the bedside table uncluttered and can be stocked in advance for patients who enjoy just being left alone for awhile.

—Keep a small pad and pencil with your supplies so you can jot down items that need to be replaced. It takes no longer to pick up six or seven items at the drug store than it does one. By keeping a comfortable inventory of supplies, you can shop when it is most convenient and avoid hurried trips at an inconvenient time.

Anyone who has managed a household or an office should be able to find step-savers, shortcuts and better and more efficient ways to accomplish the myriad of routine tasks. If you seem to be running back and forth, hunting the scissors or always running out of something, take a moment to sit down and quietly think through your motions and devise ways to streamline the work.

—Learn to delegate as many jobs as you can to someone else—family members who want to share in your patient's care—a neighbor who can pick up a few things for you on her shopping trip, or if you can afford it, hire a housekeeper or some part-time help. If you ever have to make a choice between scrubbing the kitchen floor and spending some time with your patient, forget the floor. It can wait or be washed by someone else.

The shortcuts and careful budgeting of your time will give you a small portion of the day to consider your own needs. The first of these should be your own physical health.

You must avoid over-fatigue. The dangers inherent in pushing yourself to the limits of your physical endurance range from lowering your resistance to the common cold, flu and a handful of other ills, to playing havoc with your emotional equilibrium. You may find your problem-solving ability deserting you, your frustrations mounting, you may become angry without provocation, burst into tears for no apparent reason and find depression is weighing you down. In general, you are having a difficult time keeping your emotions under control. These are all warning signs along the road to total exhaustion. You are burning out!

—First, try to get more rest. Take mini-breaks. Rather than pushing yourself to keep going several hours hoping that when everything is done you'll take a nap, take a five-minute break every hour. At the end of a ten-hour day, the accumulated fifty minutes of short rest periods will have kept you more refreshed than the same amount after you had become over-tired. Read one article in a magazine, watch a robin build a nest in the apple tree, lie flat on your back on the floor, feet in a chair, and contemplate the ceiling, telephone a friend, assume the lotus position and meditate, step under the shower.

—To help restore your emotional balance take time to review your daily goals. Make sure they are realistic. You may be expecting much more of yourself, your patient, your family, than is reasonable. Give yourself some time to handle emotional problems before they become serious upheavals. And take time to get a larger spiritual perspective in your life.

Remember that a persistent lack of energy and excessive fatigue can also be warning signs of illness. If you continue to feel tired despite all reasonable efforts to restore your energy, consult your doctor.

—Eat balanced meals, and eat regularly. Use vitamins and mineral supplements to avoid any deficiencies in the natural resources your body needs to maintain strength. Don't skip meals or fall back on the busy-day syndrome of just grabbing something out of the refrigerator that you can eat on the run. When you skip food throughout the day, besides depriving your body of badly needed fuel, you tend to overeat at dinner, a good way to add pounds you may not need.

—Sleep. You probably found with home care that sleep patterns have had to be changed and you may also find, as I did, that you can function well with less sleep than you normally had. I survived on two or three hours of sleep per night and could work all day with no sleep at all when I had to. Keep in mind that:

1. Your attitude about sleep is more important than how long you sleep.

2. You need to learn to get to sleep quickly and sleep soundly.

Lack of sleep is never a problem but worrying about lack of sleep can be. If you say to yourself, "I need eight hours of sleep every night

and I am losing my rest if I get less," you have set up a negative attitude. Don't concentrate on the sleep you have lost; think about the
sleep you've had.

Relaxation and meditation techniques are helpful in learning to
drop off to sleep quickly. If you can achieve a state of relaxation you
will find sleep overtaking you and that state of relaxation will improve the quality of the sleep you get.

The more you fuss and worry about not getting to sleep the more
you will disrupt the natural relaxation process, setting up a cyclical
pattern of worrying about not sleeping, not sleeping, worrying about
not sleeping, not sleeping well, ad infinitum. Conscious thought of
what is taking place can help break the pattern and meditation may
give you quicker results. I suggest you either get some books on the
subject or join a class in meditation training. Meanwhile, remember
that the natural tendency for insomniacs is to try to sleep longer
hours when in reality what they need is not more sleep but a more relaxed sleep. You have the responsibility for your own sleep quality. If
you can't sleep, use those waking hours constructively and don't
worry about it.

Here are other ways you can build up your emotional energy level:

—It is easy to lose your own identity in your patient's illness. Some
outside interests, brief snatches of time alone, attention to your own
appearance, all will help ensure your own self-esteem, lift you over
the futility of self-pity, anger and resentment, feelings of being
trapped, and will make you a more interesting person, better able to
care for your patient. There is nothing selfish in it, so don't add guilt
feelings to your other concerns.

—Don't give up your outside activity entirely, continue participation, perhaps to a lesser degree. If you find bridge or bowling or
church work enjoyable and refreshing, don't drop out. It isn't in
anyone's best interests for you to sacrifice all of your own activities
while you are doing home care. If you don't have some outside interest I recommend that you find something you like to do. Spend an
evening now and then at the library, visit a friend, take a course offered by community agencies or junior colleges, go to a health and
exercise club.

—Besides that you should make some provision for a little time when
you can just get off by yourself to think, to restore, to relax. It can be

as simple as a walk, or it could be an evening at a concert. Leisure time is one of the best morale picker-uppers that I know and does wonders for your energy level as well.

If another member of your home-care family is not available to stay with your patient, ask a friend, someone from your church or fraternal organization, a volunteer from a local agency, or hire someone through a nurses' registry.

—Take time to care for your own personal appearance. Manicure your nails, keep your hair neat and styled, take an oil or bubble bath at least once a day as leisurely as time permits to calm your nerves. Not only will you look better, feel better and see a boost in your morale, it will be reflected in your patient's morale, too. Include your patient in some of this. I sometimes manicured my own nails and did Larry's nails at the same time. During our relaxed beauty treatment we talked or listened to music we enjoyed.

Your clothing should be comfortable, but not sloppy. Clothing should make you feel good. This is not to suggest that you have to get all dressed up; slacks and a blouse are appropriate and can be just as attractive. Colorful combinations are cheerful, especially to a housebound patient.

—An outside job can be good therapy because it lets you function as your own individual in an environment totally free of health care (unless, of course, you happen to be a nurse). I worked full time and found that it helped me keep my perspective.

With some thought you can have time to do all you need to do and still have some moments for yourself. Some days the work load will be heavier, but by planning ahead you can usually arrange a lighter day to follow. If the whole family is coming over for a birthday celebration on Saturday evening (which means you will be doing all your routine nursing chores in advance of the party and then drawing from your reserve fund of energy for the preparations for the guests) just don't plan a major event for Sunday. Instead, plan a quiet day with some time for reading or other relaxed projects.

You are very important to the home-care project. Give yourself the same special concern and care that you give your patient. If you do, you can have one of the most joyous, rewarding, exciting and creative experiences that life provides.

Chapter VII

Don't Fear Emergencies

An emergency is a sudden crisis, requiring immediate action, generally a situation one is totally unprepared to handle. Fear of emergencies can prohibit or defeat home care.

After speaking to a group of nurses about home care, a nurse friend of mine introduced me to a patient's wife. The patient was a man in his mid-sixties who had had a stroke. Hospitalized for approximately two weeks, he was due to be released within a few days. The patient's condition was good. He suffered very little damage from the stroke, was ambulatory, alert and expressed a good attitude. Physical therapy was needed to strengthen muscles weakened by the stroke. The man was retired and would be able to convalesce at home without concern for a job. From the nurse's point of view, he was a good candidate for home care and the doctor had agreed on the date of release. The only problem was the wife wanted to have her husband sent to a nursing home. The patient wanted to go home and no one had told him of his wife's intent.

The problem basically was not the patient's physical condition, but the wife's attitude. She was afraid to have him at home. When I met with her she repeated over and over, "What would I do if something happened?" She was so gripped by fear that her decision had been made out of her emotions . . . she was afraid she would not be able to handle an emergency at home. Despite my efforts and the advice of medical staff, she made arrangements and had her husband transferred to a skilled care facility.

What bothered me about this was not her right to make the decision . . . if she felt she could not care for her husband at home, it was certainly her decision to make. The tragedy was that her decision was based on fear, and that fear changed both her life and her husband's. The nurse later told me the husband had agreed to go to the skilled care facility because he didn't want to be a burden to his wife.

This is just one example of what fear can do in a situation. You can imagine how large a role fear plays in cases where there is a high risk of emergencies and with people who need a great amount of care. My hope in writing this chapter is to free families of these fears when they want to do home care but are afraid they will not be able to handle emergencies. My own strong desire to do home care and Larry's wanting to be home overcame my fears.

Fears can stifle or defeat home care. It is important to face fears early, keeping some perspective by discussing it with your doctor and nurse to establish the validity of your feelings, and to gain the knowledge you will need to handle any emergency that arises. This knowledge will give you confidence to remain calm and to function well. Confidence develops as you determine the patient's condition, as you learn first-aid techniques to give immediate care, and as you learn about community professionals who are trained and ready to assist you.

EXPECT THE UNEXPECTED

The key to handling emergencies is to expect the unexpected. Be alert to any change in the patient's condition and ascertain when immediate action is needed. The two major areas to check are: respiration (breathing) and circulation (heart and blood supply). These two functions of the body are essential to life and any disruption in either breathing or circulation must be considered a medical emergency. The person present must give immediate, temporary assistance to the patient and telephone professionals to provide further emergency treatment. If you are alone, call immediately so help will be on its way while you do first aid. It is better to have someone else make the phone call, if possible, so that you will be able to give immediate attention to the patient.

Keep a list of phone numbers near the telephone. Don't use scraps of paper, or an address book that you'll need to find. If you have an emergency, there may not be time to look for numbers.

The numbers you should list are:
    Nurse
    Doctor

Ambulance (or Medevac Service)
Hospital
Fire Department
Police

I kept a list taped to the wall by the telephone. When an emergency occurs you will need to call immediately and even a minute or two delay can be dangerous.

Remain calm when calling. State your need quickly, precisely, and accurately. Give your address. This is not the time to go into lengthy detail. "My husband is not breathing," says it all, or "My wife fell and cut her head and I can't stop the bleeding," or "The person shows no signs of life." These statements alert the dispatcher to send the right help—fast, with red lights blinking and sirens screaming. If the situation is not as critical, it is better to call the doctor first and he will order the ambulance. Call the ambulance yourself in non-emergency cases only when you cannot reach the doctor. If the situation is not critical, state it as such—"My grandmother fell and may have a broken leg," will still bring help quickly but the ambulance can travel at normal speeds. Emergency vehicles traveling at high speeds are always in danger of colliding with other motorists. Sometimes this is necessary, but request this service only when circumstances warrant it.

The temporary care given until professional help arrives is called first aid. We have all heard the term first aid, but I don't think we realize the full significance of the importance of that initial help. It can often save a life.

There is a new movement to train lay people to handle immediate medical emergencies when professional medical people are not available or while waiting for the ambulance. In many large cities this training is not only in first aid, but is geared specifically for victims of heart attack. In many instances, first aid or cardio-pulmonary resuscitation is the victim's only hope of survival.

Cardio-pulmonary resuscitation, CPR as it is called, is a combination of artificial respiration and artificial circulation, which should be started immediately as an emergency procedure when either breathing or circulation stops.

Dr. Donald Rosenthal, internist in the San Francisco Bay Area, wrote a letter to local schools to encourage them to have faculty and students take cardio-pulmonary resuscitation training. The following are excerpts from that letter: "As you know, cardio-pulmonary resuscitation (CPR) is an established technique at the present time which has saved many lives. The indications and the methods are simple to learn; there is no liability on the part of the person performing the CPR if the subject dies, and many, many lives have been saved by the prompt use of CPR.''

Like many doctors, Dr. Rosenthal realizes the importance of having people trained to give immediate help when emergencies arise. You do not have time to call a doctor to get advice or to call an ambulance if a person is choking on food in a restaurant, or their heart has stopped. Survival depends on having someone on hand who can give immediate aid before help arrives.

The American Red Cross, many hospitals and other organizations give first aid instruction. *Everyone* should have a basic knowledge of first aid and CPR to give immediate aid in the event of severe bleeding, poisoning, burns, and shock (which accompanies many kinds of injuries and accidents.) You will learn when to move or not move a patient. Even if you have taken a first-aid course, keep an up-to-date first-aid book handy for reference. One that I would recommend can be obtained from your local American National Red Cross office.

Dr. Donald Trunkey, Chief of Surgery at San Francisco General Hospital, states, "There has been a myth over the last two decades that organized medicine and safety services alone will save your life when you're injured, have a heart attack or are in a disaster. This is a fallacy. Without a well informed public capable of immediate emergency action, all the training of professional medical people is wasted. The odds are slim that trained help can respond to a non-breathing victim in the four to six minutes he has to live without breath. Therefore, we must depend on you—the citizen—to keep the victim alive until professional help can reach the emergency." (Quoted from an article in the *San Francisco Chronicle,* Tuesday, August 29, 1978.)

In some areas paramedic services are available for help in case of emergencies. Personnel are specially trained paramedics. As each call is received, a unit is dispatched along with a fire department vehicle. The units have communication equipment linked directly to local hospitals. Information about the patient can be transmitted to hospital personnel, the hospital advises, and emergency treatment is given immediately. Paramedic organizations usually hold classes in CPR, have speakers available to educate the community in emergency procedures and provides stand-by units at community events. They do charge for their services. Check your local telephone directory to see if you have a paramedic service in your area. In case of an emergency, if you do not know the telephone number of an ambulance or paramedic unit, simply dial the operator and she will promptly put your call through to the proper agency.

Some areas are devising special three-digit emergency numbers to call for quick response. Special electronic computers record the caller's geographical location and directs the call to the proper department. Even if a caller becomes unconscious before giving the address—the lighted electronic board alerts the dispatcher to the caller's location. Even children can remember a simple number. A six-year-old boy used the number to call for help when his grandmother collapsed while she was caring for him. People living alone can get immediate aid by dialing either "O" for operator or the three-digit emergency number if their community has one. If you would like to find out if your county has a special emergency number, call your police department or telephone company business office. Notification of local police and/or fire departments that you have a bed patient in the house may assist in a future time of emergency.

Many large hospitals now have trauma centers which handle emergencies from smaller hospitals. Patients are brought by ambulance, helicopter or flying ambulance from outlying regions where they have been given emergency care but still need specially trained staff for further emergency treatment. Trauma Centers assist in disasters such as fire, collapse of buildings, air crashes, accidents involving several people, gunshot wounds and stabbings. The trauma team consists of doctors and nurses trained to handle critical patients with the greatest skill and speed. Expert doctors and nurses are on duty twenty-four hours per day and the trauma center has the most sophisticated equipment possible to save lives.

Trauma is defined as "accidental or intentional injury to a human being," by Dr. Donald Trunkey, Chief of Trauma Services, San Francisco General Hospital. "Often" he says, "patients are brought into the emergency room literally dead, meaning they have no heartbeat or respiration." The trauma teams use their skills to treat these emergencies.

Prevention

Prevention is the best approach. Readiness is next in importance to knowledge because even with the best and most careful planning, emergencies may occur. This can happen in everyday life even if all members of the family are well. You do not quit living because you are afraid "something will happen." You live fully and completely—exercising good judgment and safety precautions—and handling emergencies if, and when, they occur. That should also apply to home care.

Remember, you have the advantage of knowing the patient. You know what is normal for him. This gives you a good basis for making sound judgments when you need to make a quick decision.

Even when the patient has had a good day you cannot become complacent. Larry had been home for five months. We had survived an abscess, hallucinations and the shingles. The physical therapy had continued and Larry was beginning to show signs of strengthening and improvement. He was now able to sit on the edge of the bed holding his own legs in place, instead of having his knees tied together with one of my cloth belts. We were beginning to get him up in the wheelchair again, taking him into other rooms and outside in the warm summer air, where he could sit and view the lovely surrounding hills. We even took him for a drive one Sunday when a friend came over and helped me get Larry into the car.

The following day, after an intensive physical therapy session, which was ending just as I came home from work, Mary, Lyn and Larry showed me what he could do. I was so pleased that at long last he was showing real progress. Lyn and I discussed his care that day and Lyn and Mary left. I crawled up on the waterbed and Larry talked enthusiastically about the day. This was our time alone and we looked forward to those first few minutes of privacy each day when we could share events and bring our lives back into focus. Finally, I pulled myself off the bed and told Larry I would prepare dinner. Larry asked me to give him a pain shot so he could relax and take a little nap while I was in the kitchen. I checked the chart and he had not had any pain medication for several hours. I prepared his small dose and injected it into the hip muscle. I then turned him over into a more comfortable position so he could rest for awhile.

I checked on him from time to time while dinner cooked. He was sleeping peacefully. When dinner was ready, I went to awaken him. "I don't want to eat now," he said. "Let me sleep a little longer."

"Alright," I replied. "Maybe your therapy was too strenuous today."

When I tried to awaken him about a half hour later, he was even more sleepy. I called Lyn to ask her advice. "He's never done this before," I stated. "What should I do? Do you think he's alright?"

"Try giving him some liquids and see if that helps him," she advised. I prepared a drink in the blender. I added a raw egg because it didn't look like I was going to be able to get him to eat dinner. He drank about half a glass for me but was still drowsy. I turned on the TV for the evening news in hopes that the noise would help him be more alert. And I sat on the bed with him. When our son John came in a little later, Larry hardly responded. This was unusual. They normally greeted each other and talked for awhile.

I followed John into his room. "Come back in and look at the way Dad's breathing," I said. "Maybe I'm imagining things, but it looks to me like he's breathing more through his mouth than his nose."

We walked back into Larry's room. John walked over and took Larry's hand. He stood and watched his breathing. We both walked back into the hallway. "I've never seen him breathing like that before," John said.

"That's all I wanted to know." I picked up the phone and dialed Lyn's number. "Lyn, the liquid didn't help. He seems to be going into a deeper sleep. He's breathing through his mouth now."

"Try getting some coffee into him as a stimulant. Take his blood pressure and I'll be there in about ten minutes," she said.

I got the coffee and went into his room. I called John and the two of us got Larry into an upright position, propped up so he could drink. Larry was not helping at all now. He drank only a small portion; I could not keep him awake for any more of the coffee. The blood pressure had dropped a little but was not critical. I began massaging Larry's arms and legs and talking to him all the time I worked.

Lyn arrived and she listened to his lungs with the stethoscope. "We better call the doctor," she said. "Keep working with him while I call."

I heard her explaining in medical terms what had happened. "Donald will meet us at the hospital, he's calling the ambulance and will tell them to bring oxygen." John was listening and said he would go outside with a flashlight and wait for the ambulance. He opened the garage door so they could get right up to the door of the apartment.

I took off my robe and dressed while Lyn talked to Larry. She rubbed his arms and chest and kept saying over and over, "Come on Larry . . . wake up."

Just as I slipped my feet into my shoes I heard John's voice from the garage. "In this way," he said.

The ambulance attendant entered the room and put the portable oxygen mask on Larry's nose and mouth. "Breathe deeply, Larry," Lyn kept saying.

Since we had a narrow hallway leading into the bedroom and I knew from previous experience that we would have a hard time getting the gurney in, I started giving directions to save time. "John, get on the other side of the bed. We'll take him out on our own equipment." We lowered Larry into a flat position and lifted him off the bed on our lift board. The ambulance driver went along with the instructions. Lyn grabbed Larry's legs and we maneuvered him out the door, into the hallway, out into the garage area and onto the waiting gurney. The other attendant started rolling him toward the waiting ambulance, which already had the door open. While they were loading him into the ambulance, I grabbed my purse, and gave John the keys to the car so he could follow us to the hospital. By the time Lyn and I climbed into the ambulance, the motor was running and we pulled out of the driveway. I sat in back with Larry and one attendant; Lyn rode in front with the driver. From time to time she would look back at us and I tried to give her some indication of what was happening. The freeway was only two blocks from our home and as soon as we hit the freeway, the driver turned on the flashing light and we drove at high speed to the hospital.

"Come on, baby," I repeated. "You're doing fine now. Just keep inhaling for me." Larry looked at me and I knew he understood. "We'll be at the hospital in a few minutes and Donald will meet us there." "Just hang on! Keep breathing deeply."

I held his hand and softly kept telling him to breathe. When we pulled up at the emergency room door the doctor was waiting. He took charge.

John parked the car and joined Lyn and me in the emergency room waiting area.

"I don't understand it," I said. "He had such a good day. His therapy went well, and he was so happy when I came home."

Larry was admitted as a patient and remained unconscious for four days. Lyn and I stayed in his room, taking turns; one of us was with him at all times. We were concerned because neither intravenous solutions, antibiotics for the infection they discovered, nor the oxygen had brought him back to consciousness. Finally, the third night, Lyn decided to spend the night at the hospital with me. The doctor had arranged for a bed in Larry's room and we took turns lying down. But neither of us slept. Shortly after midnight John came in and we all three sat waiting together. About 2:00 A.M. I urged John to go home because he had the early shift at work. Lyn and I read and took turns talking to Larry, turning him and observing him for signs of change.

Just as the first rays of the morning light hit the hills across the bay, I got up from the chair and walked over to the window. Lyn had been lying down.

"It's morning . . . there's something about the way the dawn breaks that seems to give me energy," I said.

You'll need it. You have to be at work in a couple of hours," Lyn retorted.

"What about you? You have a full nursing shift here today too." We both smiled. Neither of us cared about the long hours.

"Why don't you rest for an hour and I'll watch him," Lyn said.

"Maybe I should," I replied. She got up and I took her place on the warm cot. "I think he should be turned over," I said. "Do you want me to help?"

"No, I can do it," she replied. I turned over and felt my body begin to relax. I was tired.

"WAIT" . . . When I heard Larry's voice, I bolted up from the cot and went over to the bed. Larry looked at me and at Lyn. "Why are you turning me?'' he asked. Lyn and I were both nearly hysterical with laughter. Now neither of us was tired. Larry was awake, after four long days.

"You see, Lyn," I said. "I told you I was not superstitious about it being the 13th!" It was a beautiful 13th for us!

We had had a real emergency at home. But our team effort had worked. When we brought Larry home again we knew that we'd had a close call, but we also knew our jobs. And we knew our patient; that was our strength and our hope for coping with any future emergencies—and we had help in the community.

Take advantage of that community professional help. If some situation occurs and you are in doubt as to what has happened or how to treat, *do nothing* until you get advice from a professional. No treatment is better than mistakenly given treatment. If you have taken first aid and CPR you should be able to respond appropriately in any situation.

Change (What Does it Mean?)

Life is changing, it is never static. Change can be beneficial and change can be a clue or sign of an impending problem. In these situations you have time to evaluate and treat. But you must always be alert to change!

You will have to be alert to any significant change such as high fever or low blood pressure or any symptom which you consider abnormal for your patient. This is the time to call your doctor or if significant changes happen in the middle of the night, you can always call a local hospital emergency room for advice. Staff will know if you need to act quickly, can give first aid advice, and can advise you if it's necessary to call your doctor.

I learned this lesson very soon after I began caring for Larry at home. The first significant change happened when he had been home from the hospital about a month. We had been concerned about his red blood cell count, but blood tests showed improvement. His general condition had stabilized but he gradually became weaker from being in bed so long. His good appetite began to diminish until the only food he was taking was in liquid form. We tried every means possible to get him to drink nutritious liquids, including mixtures of powdered protein drinks with eggs, mixed in the blender. We used Tang in three flavors and powdered lemonade, all of which put large amounts of fluids in his body. Cranberry juice was given daily to help keep his urine clear. Lyn and I watched him carefully. He showed no signs of acute problems but the changes were obviously denoting some problem, but what? Temperature remained normal. Blood pressure, although low, was higher than when he was in the hospital. We checked him carefully and waited. Several days passed and he became weaker and even therapy became difficult. He complained of general discomfort and could no longer sit on the edge of the bed and dangle his legs. We still had no idea of what was causing his discomfort and decline.

The next night as I was preparing him for sleep I noticed a lump appearing about six inches below where he had had pressure sores. They were now healed and looked clean. By the time I got home from work, Lyn had used hot, wet packs on the area all day. It was now obvious that he had a severe infection, with a pus pocket extending down to the swollen area. We called the doctor and he came by the next day to check. Our diagnosis had been correct, there was an infection. The doctor expressed the need for opening the area to allow drainage. We knew we would have a difficult time persuading a surgeon to come to our home. The doctor said if the pus pocket did not open at home, Larry would have to go to the hospital. Lyn and I discussed it. We knew Larry would not want to go. We agreed that we would, if at all possible, handle this one at home.

Lyn and I continued the hot, wet packs around the clock. The idea was to get the spot to open on its own. Two days later as I rubbed the area and applied a small amount of pressure to check for swelling, the thin, new skin parted and a stream of pus spurted out. The drainage continued to gush forth for over two straight hours. Needless to say, dinner was late that night. When Lyn came the next morning I told her about my experience with all the pride of a newly graduated nurse! She said I had done a fine job and I was absolutely elated that I had been able to cope with the situation. Most particularly, I was proud that our home care worked!

The doctor came to check the area. A culture of the infection determined the type of organism and what drug would be effective against it. Lab tests showed it was the same infection he had in the hospital. We gave the prescribed antibiotic. The wound drained for many more days, and finally healed again.

We had several problems with blocked catheters, but these became routine procedures. We kept two extra catheter kits on hand at all times. We carefully monitored all intake and output of liquids and could tell precisely the amount of urine he should discharge each day. We could anticipate the problem and arrange for a new catheter to be inserted whenever needed.

Catheter irrigations can help prevent infection. Check with your doctor about this. It is difficult to keep the bladder free from infection with an indwelling catheter but this may be the alternative to damp skin or urine retention.

Another unusual happening in Larry's care was when a rash developed on his left upper arm. It appeared after a very hot day and we originally thought he had a heat rash. A day or two later (again on my nursing shift!), I discovered that little blisters had appeared on top of the redness. This was no heat rash, I decided. When in doubt, I thought, get help! I placed a call to the doctor and described the symptoms to him. "Sounds like you have a case of shingles," he said. "I'll come over tomorrow and have a look." Look he did, and that is what we had. Although shingles are painful and cause great discomfort, it was another condition we could handle at home.

Home care can be the best of all possible worlds for both the patient and the family. But it does require that you be alert, ever-watchful for problems, and seek help and advice when needed.

The team effort—Lyn, Mary, the doctor, the pharmacist, our children, our friends—all working together made home care successful for us. Despite all the ups and downs—the close feeling we had for one another sustained and inspired us. These experiences taught us about changes—some temporary, some treatable at home—and some which developed into full-blown emergencies.

You need to know how to determine change. You can determine change by being alert to any deviations, either physical or emotional. Good nursing procedures can record daily norms. For instance, if you record daily temperatures or blood pressures on the chart you can establish norms. If the temperature or blood pressure changes slightly, it can indicate a problem. Urine output and bowel function are also charted and can be easily evaluated. You need to record any unusual physical or emotional symptom on the chart so you have a basis for comparison.

What does change mean? It can mean something as simple as an "off day" for patients or something as serious as a coma, or other emergency. If you cannot determine what the change means, check with the nurse of call the doctor.

When do you wait—when do you call the doctor? If the change is minor such as a rash, wait for a day or two to determine the cause or the severity. But you call the doctor whenever you have a situation you do not understand, cannot handle or if you are in doubt about its significance.

Physical symptoms of change:

Rash: may be allergy to food, medication, clothing, soap, etc. or sign of disease.

Change in temperature (fever or chills): may be a sign the body is reacting to an infection or virus.

Difficulty in breathing: can be very serious, contact the doctor immediately.

Change in blood pressure: check the blood pressure. If it increases slightly, determine the exact amount of increase. Evaluate to see if blood pressure has been aggravated due to an emotional upset. If the increase is great, or if you have any doubt about the change, call the doctor.

Sleeping more than usual: may be a reaction to one medication, combination of drugs or due to emotional stress. Sleep can be an escape. It may also be a temporary reaction to help the body recuperate (such as after surgery, when the body needs more rest in order to heal).

Sleeping less than usual: again, may be a reaction to medications or due to anxiety. Keep a careful watch on the patient's sleep habits. Call the doctor if the pattern doesn't stabilize.

Lack of appetite: can be a physical reaction to a disease or may be a sign of emotional stress. Substitute a liquid diet and soft foods. If pattern continues, call the doctor.

Skin care: check for excessive dryness, dampness or breaks in the skin. Dryness must be treated before actual breaks occur (see previous chapter on Decubitus Ulcers).

Changes in general appearance: Sometimes you will note a change in physical or emotional appearance without a specific symptom appearing. At one point, Larry's entire physical and emotional appearance deteriorated. Normally enthusiastic, he was lethargic. Usually interested in eating, he didn't care for food. This was a sign that something serious was happening. Our awareness made us alert and we discovered an internal infection. The first change in general appearance gave us a clear clue to an impending problem.

Change in mood: People normally change moods; this is a natural part of life. The expression of feelings is a healthy process, moving a person through a full range of emotions. Any change in mood may be a temporary, normal reaction to illness or injury. Allow the patient to express feelings. It is important that patients be allowed to do this. Be a good listener. Sometimes talking brings a patient into a new dimension of consciousness. Don't try to give advice in the middle of his sharing with you. Let him talk, or cry or yell. What he needs is to know that someone cares enough to listen. Continued emotional moods *not normal for the patient* should be carefully noted and you should seek professional advice from the nurse or doctor. Your contribution, as a family member, is the valuable determination of what is "normal" for the patient.

Hallucinations may be a reaction to one medication, a combination of drugs or an overload of emotion. Check with the doctor to determine if the hallucinations are medication induced. During hallucination, allow the patient to live the fantasy as long as it does not put him in any physical danger. What he sees and feels is very real to him. You can tell him honestly that you do not see or feel what he does, but don't try to get him to "return to normal." This will happen naturally under the care of the doctor. It is important that you remain calm and confident so the patient will have a solid point of reference.

We had experiences with hallucinations. During the time Larry had the infection he hallucinated. He had occasionally hallucinated before during his hospital stays. You have to know the person to know what is fantasy and what is normal regressive memory. For instance, sometimes when I knew he was hallucinating, the nurses thought he sounded perfectly rational.

One day when I arrived, Larry had a new nurse caring for him and he was instructing her to adjust the overhead trapeze bar. She was busily following his instructions and he sounded perfectly rational. He began to describe a part of the physical therapy apparatus that he had had at the special spinal cord disability center during his previous stay. There was no apparatus here that was comparable. The nurse was hopelessly confused, partly because he sounded so knowledgeable (which he was) and partly because she was not familiar with what he was describing since what he described, although logical, did not exist in the hospital. He was hallucinating. He *saw* what he described and there was no way we could convince him that we did not see what he saw. I was glad I was there to explain to her what he was describing, so she could stop trying to adjust a nonexistent piece of equipment.

Another time the staff thought he was hallucinating and I knew that his actions were normal for him. For example, one afternoon when I arrived from work, the nurse greeted me with "Mr. Baulch is really hallucinating today." "What is he saying?" I asked. "Well, he has been talking at great length about being in prison." I laughed. "He's not hallucinating." I explained. "He is an American Baptist Minister and his ministry for the past thirteen years has been in prisons. Before that, he was a prisoner at San Quentin. He is merely reliving a part of his own life." This is one way the family can help the staff; families know the patients.

At home, we had a different kind of hallucinatory phenomenon. Larry was totally rational except that at times he saw moving images in the pictures around the room. He got quite upset that we couldn't see them. He asked each and every visitor if they could see what he saw. Finally he came to the conclusion that we were all really missing something special and that he was the only one privileged to see them! Lyn and I discussed how to handle this latest occurrence and decided it would be better to be honest with him and try to keep things at home as normal as possible. We still do not know what caused his mental state—whether it was the effect of the infection itself, a reaction from the medication or a completely psychological process caused by his having to endure one more setback. But one morning about a week later, Lyn arrived and Larry smilingly announced that "there were no more films being shown on the pictures." Lyn and I laughed and knew that he had joined us fully again. You may never have this situation, but it is important to be alert to change of any type.

Change in Personality

Be alert not only for physical changes that may indicate an emergency or need for treatment, but also be aware of changes in the personality of the patient.

Some emotional expression is normal but drastic changes in emotions over a longer period of time can be a warning of physical change or they may need to be discussed with either the doctor or nurse. The more serious the illness, the more change you might encounter. You will need to care for the patient emotionally as well as physically.

If a patient becomes angry and difficult when he is in pain, this is understandable but some solution needs to be found to relieve the pain and soothe the emotions. If the patient remains hostile even when he is no longer in pain, then you will need to handle the emotions separately. You then know he is angry about something else and the anger is not pain induced.

A patient may be depressed when chemotherapy causes nausea. Normally the nausea subsides in a day or two. If the patient's personality returns to normal when the nausea disappears, you know it was normal reaction. No one likes being sick! But if the depression continues, it needs to be dealt with as a problem itself.

From a holistic view, the body, emotions and spirit are connected. All must be considered important. Emotions left unrecognized and untreated can be a serious problem in themselves, sometimes reaching emergency proportions requiring professional advice.

Some emotional warning signs are:

Negative Emotions

Negative emotions are expressions of inner conflicts. They are "I'm not OK," in Dr. Thomas Harris' transactional analysis terminology. Although negative emotions have the same center, their outward manifestation may be either active or passive.

Active negative emotions signify a certain amount of patient participation, even though it may be through frustration, criticism, pity, anger, or hatred. Patients are at least voicing a disapproval of their situation. This disapproval leaves an option open for constructive change—"I don't like what has happened to me," can be the first step to making a commitment for participation to improve either the physical, the emotional, or spiritual aspect of their lives.

Passive negative emotions are more difficult to overcome because they not only stem from "I'm not OK," but the patient has given up. He feels he is a victim, that some outside force has power over him and there is nothing he can do to change his situation.

The reality of the situation, however, is that both active and passive negative emotional states have the seed for change and that the patient can participate fully in that change. This is the value of the holistic approach to illness.

If the "I'm not OK" attitude can be seen as changeable, as an opposite of "I'm OK," patients can transcend the negative pattern. Families, too, can get into the same pattern as patients and the situation only changes as attitudes change.

NEGATIVE EMOTIONS

Active	*Passive*
frustration of dependency	depression
irritability	lack of motivation
self pity	feeling of unworthiness
hatred of life	guilt
	boredom
	overly serious-lack of humor
	hopelessness

Active Negative Emotions

The Frustration of Dependency. We are taught that growing up means to become *independent*. The more things you can do for yourself the more independent you are. When you become seriously ill, or handicapped you feel the frustration of being dependent.

Mrs. J.N. was a stroke patient. She was at home with a nurse during the day. She could walk with help, feed herself with the use of a brace on her hand enabling her to hold a spoon. Her speech was limited and difficult to understand; but her mind was clear and functional. This imbalance of a normal healthy mind and a non-functioning body caused her acute frustration. She could not communicate verbally or by writing notes as an alternative. She, like most patients, found it difficult to be in such a helpless position, feeling the indignity of having all personal needs handled by others. All of the things we take for granted, brushing our own teeth, wiping our own mouth or blowing our nose, combing our hair, putting on make-up, shaving, all had to be done for her.

The attitude of the nurse and family is important. Try to minimize all unpleasant tasks where the patient feels embarrassment. Make it routine. Carry on a light conversation about any pleasant subject that will help the patient relax and not feel centered on the problem. If possible, be humorous. It's impossible to be problem-centered when you're laughing. Be sure patients do everything they can for themselves. Reinforce the physical therapy teachings by repeating what has been learned at each opportunity. Help patients feel that their condition is changeable.

Hope is the only foundation on which patients can build. A nurse's patience will help them relax. Remind them often that they have something to contribute.

Irritability comes from a feeling of loss of control in a situation. Patients may find fault with little things, become overly critical, difficult to please. They are usually not upset with what they complain about, but are upset because they are ill or handicapped, and feel aggravated about the situation.

Self Pity: The feeling of "I'm OK" and everyone else is "OK"— ("Poor me!") This feeling shows a resignation to the situation but the pity aspect keeps it an active symptom, so long as it is expressed.

Hatred of Life and Hopeless Plight. Sometimes patients just get tired of being sick, tired of pills, tired of being cared for. They may even begin to feel that they are a burden and that their family would be better off without them.

They may hate life. They may feel cheated, deprived. Sometimes the days go on seemingly endlessly, and the condition either remains the same or it worsens. They may feel that everyone else is having a good time. This can especially be true for young people who are ill or handicapped.

They may become withdrawn or cry. The futility of trying causes depression. They feel defeated when they have a recurrence of an old illness or if some new problem develops. They may become angry. They may shout at anyone or anything.

Passive Negative Emotions

Depression. When their general disapproval of their illness moves into resignation of their condition, they may become depressed. Depression is a feeling of hopeless helplessness. They feel there is nothing they can do about the situation. Depression is a first step in giving up.

Lack of motivation is the feeling that patients have no chance to improve the situation. "What difference does it make"—"Why try."

Feeling of unworthiness. If the patients' view of themselves is one where they only feel important when they are healthy—then illness, which is the opposite of health, will make them feel worthless. If they relate totally to their job, or their family role, any serious disruption will shake their self image.

Guilt. People may feel that they let everyone down by being ill. They may feel that they are a burden, partly because they require physical care, partly because family members must adjust their lives to accommodate the care needed. Illnesses also cost money. The longer the illness, the more costly it becomes. If insurance does not cover this cost, or if the patient can no longer earn an income, this may add to the stress. Then even trivial, day-to-day problems can appear out of perspective to the patient. We are taught in our humanistic society that the ability to "produce" makes us worthwhile human beings. The "work ethic" is idolized. We feel guilty when we can no longer produce, even if we are ill. We feel that we have no value as a person if we cannot "do" something.

Boredom. Being bedridden can cause a feeling of boredom, of ennui. But it is also a stopping of our frantic need to "be busy." It gives one the time to think, reflect and truly share with another human being. Visitors are welcome and the time available for sharing can be one of the greatest blessings of illness.

At the right time, try to move your patient into a different area, out of doors if possible. Even a trip to another room helps. If they must be confined to one room, you will have a bigger problem to divert their attention to something else.

Develop hobbies, such as coin collecting, stamp collecting, reading, artwork, music, playing tapes on a subject the patient is interested in.

The art of conversation comes in handy here. Talk about some news item, some upcoming event, keep patients feeling that they are a part of the world and not shut off.

Lack of humor. In another section, I discussed the importance of humor. When patients become overly serious and do not allow humor to relieve the situation, negative emotions will take precedence in their lives. Since there is a direct link between the emotional and the physical, the use of humor is a very important healing tool.

Hopelessness is the final stage of giving up. It can be a total state of withdrawing from life—a state in which the patients are saying "There's no use trying—nothing can be done"

These attitudes, turned into the negative, can be changed. Patients are responsible for their own attitudes. It is not a problem of what happens to us—but how we feel about the situation. Our attitudes determine how full a life we have.

Hypochondria. I do not think of hypochondria as an imagined illness. I think of it rather as excessive worry or anxiety about an illness and an obsession that is out of proportion to the reality of the situation. Illnesses must always be kept in perspective and a healthy attitude maintaned.

You may not be able to call an ambulance for an emotional emergency but treatment and counseling are available.

NON-MEDICAL EMERGENCIES

There are other emergency situations which may occur. They require your being alert and taking every precaution possible to avoid their happening while you are doing home care.

Fire

According to a recent report issued by the National Fire Prevention and Control Administration, one person dies in a fire every hour. The number of fire deaths increases each year. These are primarily from deaths in residential homes. The fire department reports that the two major contributions to fire are: cooking and smoking. Extreme care should be taken when you are cooking. Never leave your home if you are using the stove. Keep the oven free from grease. Smoking in bed is most dangerous but ashes dropped in chairs, sofas, and carpets can also cause fires. Only your caution can prevent fires. Your local fire department will give you advice and assistance. Some suggestions they make for preventing fires are:

1. Be careful with cigarettes. Do not leave them lying around or smoke in bed where you might fall asleep.

2. Be sure all electrical wiring is safe. Do not repair cords or plugs with tape. Replace frayed cords.

3. Use a fire screen when fireplace is being used. Check chimney and clean as needed.

4. Eliminate flammable liquids from storage areas.

5. Remove stored trash and papers.

6. Do not leave matches or lighters where children can locate and play with them.

7. Never leave children or invalids alone in a house.

8. Install a smoke detection device to alert the family to fire.

9. Keep a fire extinguisher in a convenient place to put out small fires before the fire department arrives.

10. Keep the number of the fire department handy on your telephone list and call *immediately* if you discover a fire.

11. Inspect your house and plan for evacuation in case of fire.

12. If you have a fire do not re-enter house after everyone is out to remove valuables. Material objects are not worth risking your life to save.

Loss of Electricity

Keep flashlights and candles in convenient locations for use in a power failure. Since lights go out suddenly be sure you can find a flashlight easily. I keep one flashlight on the side of the refrigerator, held in place by a magnet. I purchased two battery operated lamps, which can be found in either discount stores or camping supply stores. I kept one in the bedroom and one in the bathroom. They are inexpensive, and provide a great deal of light.

You will need the flashlight to check your fuse box to see if the power failure is in your own home or is a local situation. Be sure you know where your fuse box is located and that you have extra fuses on hand. If you have circuit breakers, be sure you understand ahead of time how to reactivate the power. Then have an electrician inspect your home to determine why the fuses blew out or circuit breakers went out. These are signs of either a short in the wiring or an overload. Any problem must be corrected to prevent fires. If the loss of power is local, call the gas and electric company emergency repair service in your area. If your patient is on any kind of monitoring or electrical assist device, be sure and register with your local electrical company or police.

Telephone Malfunction

The telephone is essential to home care because it is the most important link with the community. Check your equipment and have any loose or frayed wires replaced. Plan ahead how you would handle a telephone malfunction. You may be able to use a neighbor's telephone to call repair service but you should also know where the closest pay telephone is located for emergency use. Always keep a dime in a compartment of your wallet or purse for this use. If you need telephone repair quickly, advise the repair service of your home care need. They will give you priority service.

Breakdown of Your Car

General maintenance at regular intervals, including replacement of tires, batteries, and other essential equipment, should keep your car in good operating condition. You may need to use your car for transporting a patient in the event of an emergency as well as for doing errands. As in all other emergency procedures, it is important to plan for contingency situations and have an alternate means of transportation, such as ambulance or taxi.

Emergencies can be handled successfully. The benefits and joys of home care are worth the challenge of dealing with change. Even if we have patients living in other kinds of care instutitions, we must be alert and ready for emergencies. Emergencies are a part of life itself. There is no safe place to hide to become crisis free—but life can be full and exciting if we accept change and are as ready as possible for all events that may happen to us.

Chapter VIII

If You Are Dealing with Pain

What is Pain?

We are all familiar with pain in some form. As children we learn the first basic lesson of pain—it hurts. Then we decide that pain is to be avoided. We know, often from experience, what we can do to avoid pain. One of our earliest memories may be of touching a hot stove. The pain, in cases like this, is a prime motivator to keep us from injuring ourselves. Pain also alerts us to a condition that needs medical attention. If we experience severe pain in some area, we go to a doctor for diagnosis. Pain thus provides a valuable assistance by giving us warning signs to recognize injury and disease. We are also acquainted with pain from minor accidents—cuts, sprains, bumps and bruises, from overexertion when muscles become stiff and achey, and from toothaches which send us rushing off to a dentist. All of these are temporary pain incidents and our salvation is knowing that with proper care on our part and immediate attention, we will return to our preferred pain-free existence.

There are injuries and diseases which cause chronic or long lasting pain. In these cases, you need more knowledge about pain, pain relieving techniques and long-term supervision by one or more physicians.

Larry, during his cancer illness, had many kinds of pain. He commented that the presurgery tests were often more uncomfortable and painful than surgery; partly because of psychological tension beforehand, and partly because unlike surgery which had the benefit of anesthesia, presurgery testing was done with little pain relief medication. Post operative pain may have been more intense but he felt it was more bearable because the surgery was over and the hope of full recovery gave him an emotional lift. He also had two spinal surgeries which were painful but with medication and other pain relieving techniques, he remained functional.

The worst pain, for him, was from the shingles. He described it as "the feeling of a hot iron being pressed against the skin of his arm." Not only was the pain itself more intense but the pain would hit at unpredictable intervals, often many times per hour, even awakening him from sleep. This disruptive pain cycle raised havoc in our lives and undermined our attempt at relaxation therapy. Medication seemed to have no effect on the pain. Fortunately, shingles only last from four to six weeks, and we did have that hope of relief. Some chronic pain, however, goes on for months and years.

How is Pain Measured?

We have thermometers to measure temperature. Two patients who have temperatures of 104 can be compared. But it is difficult to compare pain because pain is an individual experience. Therefore, doctors rely on the patients to describe where the pain is felt, when it began, the type of pain (dull ache, sharp stabbing, hot, etc.), and whether the patient has constant or intermittent pain. It is important that people evaluate their own pain and honestly tell doctors how they feel. Doctors can then test, diagnose, and treat appropriately. Attaining pain relief requires full patient communication and participation with the doctor.

Chronic pain which begins with an illness or injury can develop into a major health problem. Pain costs billions of dollars per year in medical costs, disability payments, lost work hours, and in the sales of non-prescription pain medication. Pain is responsible for more lost work hours than any other disease. Chronic pain can be a disease itself.

The Pain Cycle

I heard a lecture on the pain cycle which was helpful to me in understanding what Larry and I experienced. There are two kinds of pain: acute, which comes from an illness or injury, is short-term, and the patient will be pain-free when the illness is cured or the injury heals. In these cases, prescribed narcotics for pain relief are valid. Chronic pain, however, begins with an illness or injury but is long-term. Narcotic therapy for long-term chronic pain does not solve the problem and may create other problems. People build up a tolerance for narcotics and need larger doses to achieve the relief they formerly got from smaller doses. Narcotics can alter the patient's personality, making him "spaced out" and/or depressed. The cycle then is: you have pain, feel depressed, and take prescription narcotics for relief. Narcotics produce more depression, which causes more pain. You are back to square one, so to speak. So you start the cycle again. Some doctors prescribe "mood elevating" drugs to offset the depression caused by narcotics alone. Now you have one drug to compensate for another. This cycle could be endless unless the patient wants to break the pattern and will use some other method of pain relief or pain control when total relief is not possible. Chronic pain patients want relief but the price they pay for long-term narcotic use may prove to be too high.

Pain Treatment Centers

Pain cuts across specialized medicine divisions and intrudes in all fields of treatment. Because it is such a widespread problem and often difficult to treat, some doctors are now specializing in pain control. The number of pain centers or clinics is increasing in many cities in the United States and several university hospitals have a department for pain control. Pain centers use a "team approach," utilizing the talents and expertise of several doctors. Many doctors send chronic pain patients to a pain center for treatment. Patients may also seek the advice of pain specialists.

Doctors in the pain centers evaluate the patients in a holistic way: physical, emotional and spiritual, looking at what is happening in the patient's whole life. After a consultation, the doctors may require patients to remain in the clinic for treatment and to learn pain control techniques or they may treat patients on an out-patient basis.

ALTERNATIVE METHODS OF PAIN RELIEF OR CONTROL

Heat and Cold

Doctors may prescribe the use of either heat or cold to relieve pain. Heat and cold basically work the same; they increase circulation to the affected area. Patients should never indiscriminately choose to use either heat or cold, because the treatment could be dangerous or inappropriate for the situation. Only a doctor can determine which to use, when to use, and at what precise time intervals. Heat and cold applications provide only temporary relief and should be used only after consulting a physician.

Nutrition

When you are in pain you may not have an appetite. It is important, however, to provide the body with nutrients to maintain the balance of energy. You cannot maintain or promote health without proper nutrition. If you do not feel you can eat properly, prepare well balanced liquid meals. Vitamin and mineral supplements may be added to the diet if needed. Nutrition does not relieve pain but it strengthens the body and promotes the healing process.

Relaxation

Tenseness increases pain. Relaxation therapy is used to reduce tension for pain reduction or relief.

When Larry had cancer and I was studying books on pain, a nurse friend asked me if I was familiar with the Jacobsen technique. She said she had used it when she worked in a hospital unit for patients with burns. Burns are extremely painful and pain is difficult to relieve by medication. The more tension patients have, the more pain they have. The nurses used the Jacobsen theory of relaxation to reduce tension and to promote calmness in the patient, thereby reducing or relieving pain.

I was surprised to discover that Dr. Edmund Jacobsen's *Progressive Relaxation* was written in 1929, and that it was primarily for doctors and scientists. In 1934, Dr. Jacobsen rewrote the book for laymen under the title *You Must Relax*. In this book, Dr. Jacobsen describes his scientific study of tension and relaxation which began in 1908 in the laboratory at Harvard University. He had to overcome the general idea that relaxation meant "amusement, recreation or hobbies." Dr. Jacobsen defines relaxation as "letting go or taking it easy." "To be relaxed," he says, "is the direct physiological opposite of being excited or disturbed."

It reminded me of a "Peanuts" cartoon I saw. Lucy was sitting in a booth with a sign on the front which stated "The Psychiatrist is in." Charlie Brown stopped to tell her his problem. She listened attentively and in the last caption she gave her advice, "Relax, 25¢ please."

The advice to relax is given easily—the application is more difficult and must be learned. Doctors once prescribed "bed rest" for patients, assuming that if the patient were confined to bed they would naturally relax. They discovered that merely lying down did not guarantee relaxation. Often the minds of the patients were active— and the mental stimulation caused physical tenseness. Emotions such as fear, worry, anxiety, frustration, and anger produce physical counteractions.

Dr. Jacobsen used fine platinum wires inserted just under the surface of the skin to measure electronic impulses. Recently, scientific study with more sophisticated electronic biofeedback equipment has proven that any mental imagery of action or any emotion expressed in thought is reproduced in the body—even if the person is lying absolutely still and apparently motionless.

People do not know how to relax. They must learn a relaxation procedure. To *try* to relax often causes the very tension you are trying to relieve. Dr. Jacobsen outlines a procedure for relaxation beginning with the person lying down and progressing to learned relaxation states while in a sitting position. The goal is to learn to relax at various times of the day, even while working. It is far better to relieve tension at intervals during the day than to accumulate stress and "relax" for one hour. Dr. Jacobsen writes in detail about the various illnesses caused by tension such as high blood pressure, colitis, coronary heart disease, angina, neurological disease, asthma, insomnia, tension headaches, nausea. He theorizes that if you can relax your body totally the mind and emotions also relax. In other words—you *begin with the physical* to restore balance to the mental and emotional. Other theories are being set forth whereby *you begin with the mind* to restore order and balance to the physical and emotional. All theories agree that there is a connection between the physical and mental or emotional states.

Although relaxation is widely written about today, the study of relaxation is not new. Between 1910 and 1958, Dr. Edmund Jacobsen wrote sixty-five articles and books on his studies of relaxation.

Herbert Benson, M.D., Associate Professor of Medicine at the Harvard Medical School and Director of the Hypertension Section of

Boston's Beth Israel Hospital, begins his book *The Relaxation Response* with a quote from a Chinese physician written more than 4,600 years ago describing the connection of emotions to the physical body. Dr. Benson evaluates the present predicament of mankind and offers the Relaxation Response as an alternative to stressful living.

The book contains the "social readjustment scale" devised by Drs. Thomas H. Holmes and Richard H. Rahe, psychiatrists at the University of Washington Medical School. The chart lists events (both good and bad) and designates the amount of stress derived from each. The chart was devised after interviews with 394 individuals. We would expect so called "bad" events to cause stress, but often we are unaware that so called "good" events also cause stress. For instance, we might expect the death of a spouse to rate the highest on the scale—100, followed by divorce at 73, marital separation at 65, jail term at 63, death of a close family member at 63; but would you expect marriage to be designated at 50, with a higher stress value than being fired from a job rated at 47? Would you expect sex difficulties and gaining a new family member as being at the same level of 39? This stress chart can help you better evaluate your own life circumstances, and help you become aware of your own stress level.

In his book, *The Relaxation Response,* Dr. Benson also contributes a scientific study of medication and its effects on the physical body. He eloquently describes the history of eastern and western thought, both religious and nonreligious, and carefully outlines his "relaxation response." His theory, is that *by beginning with a change in the mental state, you can bring about changes in the physical body.*

Books, articles and newspaper stories are appearing more frequently these days about relaxation and the benefits to the person who learns relaxation techniques. Doctors and scientists are researching the body's response to stress, the biological and physiological changes that take place and the reversal of those responses when relaxation techniques are used.

The first problem, of course, is to realize that you are *not relaxed.* We think we are relaxed. We ought to be relaxed: we go on vacations and we sit in front of the television set doing nothing strenuous and we assume this is relaxation.

Non-activity does not assure relaxation.

Some people think work is strenuous and that being away from work is relaxation. Work-oriented people may feel relaxed on the job, and stressful about leisure time. What is stress to one person will be another person's relaxation. Doing yard work or tending plants is literally work for me. I do not do it well and I do not enjoy it. To me, it's stress. My mother, on the other hand, enjoys being out of doors, likes caring for plants, and enjoys watching them grow. For her, yard work is relaxation. I enjoy driving a car. I like the movement of the car itself, the mobility it gives me, the change in scenery it provides, and the exhilaration of air flowing through the car windows. Others do not like to drive and feel stress when driving, especially on crowded freeways. I enjoy speaking to groups of people and find the group exchange enjoyable. Other people might feel stress if they had to stand up in front of an audience and speak, no matter how well they knew the subject. Planning meals for guests is stressful for me, while others enjoy the culinary arts. Are these just individual differences? I believe they are personal stress areas.

That brings us to the point of understanding what stress is for us, and what then is the opposite of stress. Relaxation. If you don't recognize your stress situation, perhaps the best way to learn to identify stress is to first learn what relaxation is, then the opposite would be stress. There are many relaxation techniques and meditation courses that teach what relaxation is, and how to achieve it. You can then learn to live more calmly even under the most stressful situations. You will also learn how to empty out all the accumulated stress and hopefully learn not to accumulate stress in any form.

Stress is not physical, but it has effect on the body. Stress is emotional and is whatever causes us to feel uncomfortable, tense and nervous. That could be anything from mild anxiety to total panic. It could be frustration, anger or hostility. It could be boredom, or the feeling of monotony. It could be the pressure of time . . . having to get things done on a rigid time schedule.

Stress is being overly concerned with any aspect of your life. It's concern about your marriage, or not having a marriage; having to make decisions or worrying that you'll make the wrong one; it's seeing other people on your job getting promoted when you wanted the job, or not having a job; it's anxiety about how your children are turning out; it's worry about an older person in your family; it's trying to live on retirement income when the cost of living keeps going up; it's trying to make financial ends meet or having money and being concerned that it will all be taken away in inflation; it's concern about personal relationships; it's anything that makes you feel tense and unsure about yourself or your ability to handle the situation. The degree may vary, but it's stress.

There is piled-up stress. One stress on top of another, day after day, collected and accumulated in your head until there is no more storage room and the lid blows off like a pot that boils over on the stove. Can you imagine what your house would look like if you never emptied the garbage and trash that collects? We hire a garbage collector to carry it away, but we pay little attention to the garbage that collects in our heads.

We become so used to stress that we think it is normal and uncontrollable. That's the way life is, we say. Our bodies react to this kind of pressure and our society has a high rate of heart attacks, cancer, ulcers, colitis, hypertension, strokes, and headaches (big over-the-counter drug business to relieve you of these.)

These diseases are symptoms which indicate that some part of your body is not functioning well and you will begin treatments to see if the medical profession can undo damage that might have been prevented. And if you are a worrier, you will have a new worry: Are the treatments working? Will you recover? If you haven't recognized earlier warning signs of stress, serious breakdown in bodily function may force you to face what is happening in your life that is making you ill.

The idea of stress and its effect on the body was first developed by Hans Selye, as a nineteen-year-old medical student at the German University of Prague. In studying the cases of five patients he discovered that despite their differing symptoms, they all suffered from depleted energy, were listless, haggard and drawn. When he asked for permission to study the syndrome he could only describe as "just being sick," the young student was coldly turned down.

But he continued to work on his theories and now, in his 70s, is dean of stress research. Known as "Dr. Stress," he is founder of the International Institute of Stress on the campus of the University of Montreal. He expounds on the theory that the best way to handle stress involves taking a different attitude on the events in one's life. He believes that by perceiving events as pleasant rather than unpleasant one converts negative stress into positive stress which he called "*Eu*stress," using the Greek prefix for "good."

There is no way to live without stress, but stress can be recognized and our attitudes about stress can be changed. We can also change our attitude toward the events in our lives and change life patterns that create negative stress.

The quality of life depends on your own attitude.

Biofeedback

Biofeedback is an accepted scientific device that proves there is, indeed a connection between our mind and our body. Early forms of electronic equipment used small wires inserted under the skin to monitor relaxation, muscle tension, and nerve response. Newer equipment used today has small pads which are attached to the skin.

One of Larry's visiting physical therapists brought with her a portable biofeedback machine. Small electrodes were attached to his body. Biofeedback machines measure physical and mental activity by flashing lights, ticking noises, or written graph analysis. Our machine "ticked." We could hear ticking when the machine was hooked up.

Larry was asked to image a calm, serene scene; a lake, river, beach, forest—any place in which he felt a state of relaxation. He was then asked to inhale deeply, and exhale slowly. (This is an especially good respiratory exercise for bedridden patients who tend to breathe shallowly. Deep breathing improves oxygen content to the brain and makes the patient more relaxed.)

As Larry began the breathing exercises, the ticking began to slow down. The therapist, in a soft voice, guided Larry into both peaceful mental imagery and proper breathing to encourage relaxation. After a few minutes Larry could relax to the point that the machine was totally quiet. The machine would begin ticking immediately if he moved so much as a finger. It also ticked if Larry even mentally pictured himself doing some physical activity. So we quickly learned the importance of coordinating the mental relaxation with the physical deep breathing.

We had been using meditation for pain control but the biofeedback monitoring helped Larry improve the quality of relaxation.

Besides monitoring relaxation techniques, biofeedback is being used to evaluate brain wave action to determine states of consciousness, to train patients to control bodily functions such as blood pressure, temperature, and digestive processes. Biofeedback makes many contributions to scientific medicine but one of the greatest is by giving patients an opportunity to actively participate in their own recovery.

Breathing

In order to function well and be alert we need a sufficient oxygen supply to the brain. We all get lazy and breathe shallowly, reducing

the oxygen intake we need. Some simple exercises or walking outdoors can increase oxygen flow. Yoga exercises are particularly helpful in developing good breathing habits, if you are willing to take a
few minutes each day for practice.

Correct breathing assures your entire body of proper oxygenation.
Simply inhaling deeply to the count of three, holding your breath for
three counts and exhaling slowly for three counts (repeated three
times) will prove a powerful reliever of tension and will provide new
energy for the body.

Breathing exercises can help patients relax and fall asleep quickly,
and can quickly relieve muscle tension for simple pain relief. Used as
a supportive therapy to other techniques for chronic pain, breathing
exercises can prove beneficial.

Simple exercises may be practiced by patients, such as walking and
deep breathing. Other methods require trained therapists to teach the
patient proper use of respiratory exercise.

Meditation

Meditation is a voluntary process to achieve an altered state of consciousness. The brain has two hemispheres: the left, which is the
thinking, analytic, logical, so-called masculine side and the right,
which is receptive, intuitive, experiential, symbolic and so-called
feminine side. We live most of our lives using the left hemisphere and
leaving the power and energy of the right side untapped. Meditation
puts you in touch with the right side of consciousness. It is in the
right hemisphere that mental imagery takes place. Meditation is the
vehicle that takes you to the area of consciousness where images
form. The meditation process guides the imagery.

In an article published August 29, 1978 in the *National Enquirer,*
Dr. Elmer Green, director of the voluntary controls program at the
Menninger Foundation in Topeka, Kansas, said, "Guided imagery
does work on arthritis. It is a valid technique and is being used by
many members of the Biofeedback Society of America. They have
seen striking results . . . it isn't just in your head. The results are in
the body and can be recorded when patients are wired to a biofeedback machine."

Also giving his comments on the usefulness of imagery in controlling pain, Dr. Irving Oyle, teaching associate at the University of California Extension at Santa Cruz, said "It is the most effective pain

reliever I know of. It really works on any kind of pain, from tension headaches to pain from muscles, joints and even from terminal cancer.'' (*National Enquirer* article, November 14, 1978)

Other therapists have reported successful use of guided imagery in treating patients with rheumatoid arthritis, insomnia, migraine headaches, and for pain relief. Patients are asked to visualize what is causing their pain, an object like a knife (for stabbing pain) or a hot iron, or a heavy object pressing on some point. They are then told to visualize the object being removed and being replaced by a soft object for the heavy one, a cool object for a hot one or a smooth object for a sharp one. The idea is to replace a negative object with a positive one.

Guided imagery can bring successful results but should not initially be attempted without the training of a doctor or counselor.

Hypnosis

Hypnosis is now used as a pain killer in dentistry, obstetrics, surgery, and with terminal illness. Hypnosis can be performed successfully only with the complete consent of the patient. Like guided imagery, hypnosis operates out of an altered state of consciousness. Self hypnosis is possible after patients become trained in the technique. It is believed that pain relief occurs because it is impossible to concentrate on two ideas at once. If patients think about pain, the pain increases. When the mind centers its attention on another idea, the pain is still there but the mind does not recognize the pain. Hypnosis is one of the therapies being used by doctors as an alternative to anesthesia for patients who cannot tolerate normal anesthesia and for pain control.

Acupuncture

Acupuncture, the insertion of acupuncture needles into the body at designated points to relieve pain, is used as an anesthesia and for stimulation of organs. Acupuncture has been used for approximately 3,000 years in many countries of the world, China being the most well-known, having been used as an anesthetic there for hundreds of years. Reports of successful pain relief encouraged western doctors to explore the eastern procedure. Acupuncture is now being used for pain relief by doctors trained in its application.

Acupressure

Acupressure uses the same points that are used in acupuncture; however, instead of needles being inserted, pressure and massage are applied over acupuncture points and meridians. The theory is that energy is being blocked, and massage or pressure will release the energy flow.

TNS (Transcutaneous Nerve Stimulator)

Electronic devices are used for pain relief. TNS pads are placed over tender acupuncture points and electronic stimulation is applied. Sometimes the stimulation is applied directly to the painful areas and at other times to a related acupuncture point. Some patients may experience immediate pain relief. This therapy has been successful for some patients who had previously been unable to obtain pain relief from other treatment.

You will need a physician's order for this unit and a physical therapist will be able to instruct you in its use.

Some clinics and hospitals have trial units for patients to use for a short time in order to determine if they will be successful in pain control. This will save you purchasing a unit if it does not give you the relief for which you are looking.

Psychic Transfer

Larry and I successfully used this method. Pain can be transferred from one person to another. Both people go into a meditative state, and visualize the pain leaving the patient's body and entering the body of the other person, who sends energy and vitality into the patient. The transfer leaves the patient free for a short period of time (one to three hours in our case). The person receiving the pain then mentally releases the pain, which is relatively easy because there is no organic cause. The patient gets pain relief without the use of narcotics. This procedure is a form of guided imagery and can be learned as part of the meditation technique. Until you have been successful with imagery, you should not attempt a pain transfer. The person receiving the pain will discover it is very real—it does hurt—and you must be able to successfully release it. When done properly, it can be a good alternative to prolonged narcotic use. It is not a substitute for other treatment but can be used in conjunction with other treatment.

We stumbled on this idea by accident. Larry always teased me about being a "bundle of energy." "Don't you ever get tired?" he asked. "No, I really don't," I said. "I wish I had some of your energy," he said, laughingly. "Here, let me give you some of mine," I said. I sat down on the side of the bed. I linked our arms, wrists touching. "Now, I am going to transfer energy into you and you're going to release pain out to me," I said.

"I don't want you to have my pain," he said, pulling away. "Come on, let's try. If I get your pain, I can handle it. I haven't had any pain in my body and can get rid of it. You have it all the time. You need my energy." I connected our arms again.

"Think of a conveyor belt, my energy is coming into you, your pain is emptying into me." I repeated this over and over. I mentally thought about energy going in and pain coming out. We both had our eyes closed to help the imagery. Suddenly I felt a sharp stabbing pain in my chest, coming in from my back. I was surprised at its intensity. "You know, my pain has gone," Larry remarked. "And I do feel better." "Yes, and I know where the pain went!" I then described what I felt, it was exactly where he had had the pain. What had started out as a joke turned into a pain relief routine for use. Each time we did it, the pain would be different. Sometimes it would be sharp, sometimes a dull ache. And it would affect more than one area. Larry always confirmed what I described. There were times that I needed to take pain medication myself to get rid of the pain. Now I know how to get rid of it using meditation instead of medication, but at that time this was unknown to me.

Psychic Healing

Psychic healing, known as the "laying on of hands" is not new but is now becoming more widespread. "Laying on of hands" took on a negative connotation because of evangelists' religious application; the scientific community frowned on it as illogical and superstitious. It is ironic that new scientific discoveries have proven that the body is made up of energy. Healers' hands have a special kind of energy flowing from the fingers which can be recorded with special photographic equipment. College classes taught by nurses and doctors are now being offered, using this method. Dr. Thelma Moss, at the University of California, Los Angeles, has done a great deal of research on psychic healing and parapsychology, bringing it out of the realm of the occult into the laboratory.

Dolores Krieger, Ph.D., R.N., a professor at the Graduate School of Nursing at New York University, was one of the speakers at the first Congress of Nurse-Healers held in San Francisco in June, 1977. The meeting was attended by approximately nine hundred persons representing schools of nursing, staff from hospitals and those in private practice. Following her appearance at the congress, she gave a lecture and workshop at a local seminary, which was open to the public.

Her morning lecture was given to the entire group of conference participants. The afternoon was devoted to workshops, and I selected her workshop on Therapeutic Touch. She described the energy fields within the body and how a nurse (or family member) can be trained to either pass their hands over the body of the patient (approximately two to three inches above the skin) or by touching to promote healing. The nurse will be in a meditative state, totally free of outside stimuli. As a sensitivity is developed, the nurse can feel heat around the area where there is disease. Healing energy is then deliberately channeled to that area of the patient. The workshop included slides depicting her approach to using the meditative state for healing, and practical demonstrations involving workshop members. She outlined the transfer of energy, the role of the nurse as healer, and the art of nursing in relation to modern technology.

Whether for pain transfer, relaxation, nursing care or as an expression of love, touching was indeed a healing process, for both Larry and for me.

Whether for pain transfer, relaxation, nursing care or as an expression of love, touching was indeed a healing process, for both Larry and for me.

Surgery for Pain Relief

Surgical pain blocks should be considered only after careful diagnosis, consideration of other alternatives and complete awareness of both the desired effect of the surgery and a full knowledge of possible damage of nerves which may effect function. There are several kinds of surgical procedures including the injection of alcohol to destroy the nerve itself or surgical severance of the nerves. Some doctors believe that in cases of terminal illness, pain relief may be more desirable than impaired mobility. But the seriousness and permanence of this kind of surgery requires careful consideration.

Addiction

Pain relief is needed for patients to continue living with pain. Prescribed medications—tranquilizers, sedatives for sleep and narcotics are sold by the millions each year. Pain can often last for years, and if patients continue to take drugs over a long period of time, there is a danger of addiction. Then patients have two problems: pain and addiction. And add to this the possibility of the use of alcoholic beverages in combination with drugs and you have added another danger, death. Many doctors do not feel addiction is a problem. But patients' families, who see their loved ones deteriorating from narcotic use, would prefer another alternative. And patients hear grim stories of being hooked on prescribed drugs.

Many celebrities have died from drugs or a combination of drugs and alcohol. Their deaths are widely publicized and bring attention to the problem. Many non-celebrities die, too, with the same problems. Those who die are a posthumous witness to the lethal power of drugs. Some people who have been able to recognize their addiction in time have survived. Betty Ford had prescribed tranquilizers for pain and got into trouble by drinking alcohol while taking medication. Jerry Lewis recently admitted that he almost committed suicide because he had had 13 years of pain and was addicted to a narcotic prescribed for pain due to a back injury he sustained. Both Betty Ford and Jerry Lewis were successfully treated for their addiction.

I believe addiction can develop as a result of total reliance on tranquilizers and narcotics for long-term chronic pain. Professional help for addiction can be obtained from drug detoxification centers, and pain centers.

Placebo

The placebo in pain relief is studied to find out why patients get pain relief from pills which have no pharmacological content. When the discovery was made that the placebo worked, it was first assumed that this was entirely psychological—induced by the patient's belief in the pill as a pain reliever.

Further studies produced a new theory: "University of California researchers, exploring the realms of human pain, believe that they have found out why some people get relief from the mere act of taking medicine—even when the 'pain killer' should have no medical effect at all.

"A team from the University of California School of Medicine at San Francisco reported yesterday that in some patients the ingestion of an inert placebo triggers a series of events in the brain, which ends with the release of the body's own natural pain killers.

"The natural substances, discovered only three years ago, are called endorphins, meaning *the morphine within.* They appear to act like morphine in suppressing pain.

"Scientists have long observed that about one-third of all patients actually get relief of pain when they are given placebos—sugar pills or other inert substances that are often administered to control groups in tests of effects of new drugs.

"The phenomenon had been written off simply as a psychological one, but the researchers said that the suppression of pain was a real effect.

" 'Anything psychological involves the firing of nerve cells in an electro-chemical event,' Dr. Howard Fields said. 'Something the patient has in his body makes the placebo work.

" 'The pain is real,' he said, 'and the fact that you get relief from a placebo depends on your expectation of getting relief. So to that extent, it may be psychological. But the pain suppression is real.'

"The team, which also included Drs. John Levine and Newton Gordon, presented their findings at an international congress in Montreal. They said they had theorized that the positive effect of placebos might be the work of endorphins. They undertook a year long study with tests involving placebos, morphine and a drug called naloxone, each administered experimentally to 50 volunteer patients who had teeth pulled.

"Earlier research showed that naloxone seems to have no effect of its own on pain, but it blocks the painkilling effects of narcotics and is used to treat heroin overdoses. As expected, some of the patients— 36%—reported pain relief after injection with placebo. However, when followed up with naloxone, the effect of the placebo disappeared. The researchers concluded that relief of pain by placebos must be due to some chemical released in the brain—presumably, endorphin—that can be blocked by naloxone.

"However, why some persons respond to placebos, by releasing endorphins, and others do not, remains a mystery."

(From an article in the *San Francisco Chronicle,* "How Placebos Work," Tuesday, August 29, 1978, page 14)

The University of California is not the only test center for the placebo. Many medical colleges and hospitals are doing similar research on the placebo. The discovery of endorphin, the body's own natural opiate, could be a real breakthrough in pain relief.

Pain Games

In an early chapter I discussed games. Pain games are ones centered on pain, which can change the personality and behavior of patients, affecting all those with whom they come into contact. What person would be insensitive enough to argue with patients in pain—or bring up a problem—or make any demands on them? Sometimes patients develop a new lifestyle. They like not working and collecting disability insurance; they like having the attention of their families and they enjoy the freedom a lack of responsibility gives them. It is difficult to treat patients to make them pain-free when they get a "pay off" from their pain. They may complain about the hurt, and the hurt is real; but they do not want to give up what for them are definite benefits. In cases like these, professional counseling is needed. Without help patients will continue to play the pain game. They do not need to go back to their old job if they didn't enjoy it—and they could have better relationships with family and friends. But they must be aware of the potential of a new pain-free life.

Dr. C. Norman Shealy in his book, *The Pain Game,* writes about games patients play, games doctors play, and describes new methods of dealing with pain using his experiences with patients at the Pain Rehabilitation Center in La Crosse, Wisconsin. Although some of the book is technical, this is a must book for all patients in pain—from those just beginning the pain cycle to those who have been considered hopeless by the many doctors they have seen on their endless search for pain relief. It is also a book families should read to help them understand the pain game before their lives end up in quarrels, unhappiness and divorce. You can read this book in about three hours. It is well worth the investment of your time and may help change your attitude about pain—the first step to real relief.

Attitude

Attitude, how patients feel about pain, can limit their lives. Many pain-ridden patients live full lives because their attitude enables them to continue their activities and experiences. Others give up and let the pain dictate the kind of life they live. Doctors can treat the pain but only patients can change their own attitudes.

Larry had a lot of pain. But his psychological and theological perspective on pain and illness balanced out the physical effect. His personality transcended the pain and we were able to live a normal life. That did not mean we had the same kind of life we had before—that was not possible. But the *quality* of our life remained unchanged and we had love, humor, and strength to sustain us. Most importantly, we were able to experience it all—together.

Chapter IX

Care for the Handicapped

Home care as described in the chapter The Team Effort is applicable to people with handicaps. The goal of home care for the disabled is to encourage patients to resume their participation in the world, i.e. with their job, recreation, education and social life.

Some people are born with a physical disability or deformity. They learn early to live their lives to the fullest. It may be harder for people who are born with full healthy bodies to readjust their lives when they have an illness or injury. They may center on their loss rather than what they have left. If they feel they are complete persons without the use of the whole body, their lives can be productive and happy.

Any disease can leave a part of the body damaged. Injuries occur in a variety of ways and may leave people with different degrees of impairment.

Some diseases that disable are: emphysema and other respiratory diseases, cystic fibrosis, diabetes, amylateral sclerosis (commonly known as "Lou Gehrig's disease"), muscular dystrophy, multiple sclerosis, poliomyelitis, streptococci infections, complications from childhood diseases, arthritis, cancer, and strokes resulting from heart disease. Pain can be disabling, too.

Injuries cause impairment, paralysis and/or loss of limbs. Perinatal injury may result in cerebral palsy. Some brain injuries cause epileptic seizures. Loss of speech, hearing and sight are also disabilities. Brain damage may cause mental dysfunction. Some injuries and birth defects require reconstrucive or cosmetic surgery. Cleft palate requires reconstructive surgery, for instance. Reconstructive or cosmetic facial surgery makes a great contribution to the wholeness of people's lives.

This was demonstrated when Rudy Miller, environmental reporter for a San Francisco television station, was bitten by her dog. Her lips were damaged and she required plastic surgery. This kind of facial damage could have ended her career and totally disrupted her life. After surgery, she returned to air a program entitled "I Am Whole Again," based on stories of peoples' experiences with cosmetic and reconstructive surgery. She interviewed Amanda Blake, TV actress, who had surgery after cancer of the mouth, a woman who had breast reconstruction, a man who had his entire scalp replaced after an auto accident, and a child with an ear reconstruction. After the physical reconstruction many patients need counseling to heal the trauma of emotional wounds.

Some miraculous recoveries have been made despite grim diagnoses, but other patients have had to deal with permanent damage, living their lives in a different manner than they would have had the accident or illness not occurred.

In a previous section I wrote about physical, occupational and speech therapy. Professionals who work in these fields make tremendous contributions to patients with disabilities. They not only treat and counsel the patient and family but can advise about making the home functional for home care. Even in an institutional setting, patients have the opportunity to reevaluate their lives and make plans for new directions. But the home provides the most normal environment for that new life. The therapists can advise families on how to readapt the home, and what equipment is needed. Adjustments not only need to be made in the physical environment but in the emotional as well. How patients and families feel about their new lives is critically important.

Patients and families are afflicted by the stereotyped image that the handicapped are deficient—less than normal. But "the handicapped" are people. Their common experiences may lump them in a group, which is labeled, but that group is made up of individuals—people who have private lives, hopes, dreams and capacities for giving. If they can be thought of as individuals, rather than as a needy, helpless group that must be supported by the "healthy" members of society, our community will be enriched. I never thought of Larry as handicapped. In a wheelchair or out, to me he was the same person he always was, only our circumstances were different.

Stories of people overcoming handicaps are repeated over and over in newsi apers and magazine articles and movies. These are stories of people—individuals—who have not only survived tragic circumstances, but have a new and exciting commitment to life. Their lives take many forms and their interests are diverse, but they all contribute not only to themselves, but to their families and society as a whole. The following stories of people are taken from media sources listed in the bibliography at the end of the book.

Jim Brunotte was a cowboy in a rural California area before he went to Vietnam. He came back with one arm, two legs and an eye missing. Larry and I read about him in a newspaper. Larry called him and asked if we could help with his project, the building of a recreation ranch for the handicapped, which included a pool, trails for wheelchairs, and special horseback riding facilities. Jim continues to ride horses, for pleasure and in competition.

Clayton Turner also lives in California. He was injured when he dove into an irrigation ditch where all the local young people swam. The injury caused Clayton to be paralyzed from the neck down. At sixteen his mother put a pencil in his mouth and a piece of paper on a magazine in front of him. Now in his forties, he has gained recognition from his outstanding paintings of the Old West. "I don't know what the worst thing in the world is," he said in a recent newspaper interview, "but I know one thing, it's not being without your arms and legs."

Joni Eareckson was young, lovely, active—enjoying a summer of fun and activity before going off to college in the fall. She and her sister went swimming one warm day in the waters of the Chesapeake Bay. Joni hit bottom when she dove in and became quadriplegic. Her autobiography written with Joe Musser is a story with many facets. It begins on the bottom of the Chesapeake Bay, follows Joni through seemingly endless hours of medical treatment, clearly maps her emotional ups and downs, and graphically describes her spiritual pilgrimage. It is a classic case of the limitlessness of the human spirit, brilliant testimony that we are more than our bodies. Joni proves that there is life without the use of arms and legs. Instead of centering on her loss she centers on what she has left. . . her eyes, her hearing, her mind, and her spirit. As part of her physical and occupational therapy she learned to write by holding a pencil in her mouth. One of her letters is printed in the book and I must admit, ashamedly, that her writing is much neater and prettier than my own! Joni was interested in art before her accident and she learned to do indescribably beautiful drawings. Her art work has been displayed in art shows and she has appeared on many national television programs. Her story is a triumph, not only for herself but for those around her, her family, friends, medical staff, and therapists . . . who cared about her and supported her efforts. Life is limited only by the limitations we impose in our minds. Joni has no limitations. She lives and works and her life has purpose.

Bob Hall, a polio victim at age one, found that winning the wheelchair marathon was not enough stimulation so he entered the Boston Marathon and competed against runners. He completed the 26 miles and 385 yard course, ahead of about half the competing field.

Harry Cordellos is blind. At age twenty-one he went with a group of students from the California Orientation Center for the Blind for a weekend outdoors at a reservoir. At the time, he was depressed, timid, lacked confidence, and had almost no will to live. But that day in 1958 changed his life. Someone persuaded him to try waterskiing. He failed to get up on the skiis the first day, but the second day he stood up and glided over the water. That experience opened up a whole new life for Harry. He decided to try other things, to take charge of his own life, even though well-intentioned friends and counselors advised against his new-found determination to participate in sports.

Harry is now forty years old. He still likes waterskiing, is a competitive diver from the three-meter board, does alpine and cross-country skiing, and is an accomplished runner. He competes in many races, and in 1975 set a record for blind racers in the Boston Marathon. While running, he needs a guide who paces him. He just keeps one hand lightly on the guide's arm as they run.

He is employed as an information clerk for the Bay Area Rapid Transit Company. He wrote a book in his free time. He has a masters degree in Physical Education, but has not had a chance to teach because of his blindness. But he has used his own physical ability and personal strength to set a high standard for other blind people.

Don Klosterman was a professional football player. In 1957, during the off season, he went skiing. He had an accident on the slopes and suffered multiple injuries that left him paralyzed. When a doctor diagnosed him as never being able to walk again, Klosterman fired him. He began physical therapy, determined to be able to walk. After months of therapy he stood at the altar and was married. He returned to professional football in 1960, working first in a managerial position with the San Diego Chargers, became general manager of the Houston Oilers and Baltimore Colts and eventually worked for the Los Angeles Rams. He now successfully plays golf—his only handicap being the "strokes" he gives to other players.

David Clements, age twenty, was pronounced dead on arrival at a hospital in New York after an auto accident. An orderly found a trace of life, and immediate action on the part of the medical staff saved his life. He was in a coma for four months. When he awakened he discovered he was paralyzed on one side and could not speak. But he was determined to resume his life and go to college. Physical and speech therapy were begun and he is now a college student in Florida, has a new gruff voice, and walks with a cane.

George Covington, whose eyesight is so bad he's considered legally blind, is a photographer.

Rhea Zakich, lost her voice and her ability to communicate after throat surgery. In a desperate effort to communicate she designed a game with dice and cards. The object of the game is to have some players listen and the others share feelings. The cards are specially designed with questions to open areas for discussion. Rhea wrote her answers but could participate by listening while others verbally answered questions. Her "Ungame," as it is called, is now a commercial venture.

Richard Schultz has been a bedridden paraplegic for over thirty years. But a small Illinois town depends on him. He is the emergency dispatcher. He handles 50 to 150 calls per day for fire, police and medical units.

Irene Van Lint, of La Jolla, California, suffered an injury in an automobile accident. A subsequent blood clot caused brain damage, speech loss, and paralysis. After months of hospitalization including rehabilitation therapy, a program of occupational therapy was instituted. She began typing with one finger (with special equipment to support her arms) in an effort to communicate with her family and nurses. She wrote a book, a five-year project, entitled *My New Life,* chronicling her story and describing the support from her family and medical staff.

The first doctor I met who worked in a wheelchair was Dr. Glenn Reynolds. As mentioned earlier, when Larry was in the spinal cord disability unit at the Santa Clara Valley Medical Center, Dr. Reynolds was the head of the department. Paralyzed by polio, he wheeled into the hospital and saw patients each day. Larry said it would be hard to feel sorry for yourself when you sat face to face with a doctor who was also in a wheelchair. Just his appearance in the ward made an impact on the patients.

Dr. Duncan Holbert, also a polio victim, has a dermatology and allergy practice in Santa Cruz. He has practiced for twenty-five years, seeing patients from his iron lung. He has a staff to carry out orders but is really the one who runs the office, staffers say.

Ed Roberts is paralyzed and spends some time each day in an iron lung. Handicapped? Hardly. He was Governor Jerry Brown's choice to be Director of the California Department of Rehabilitation. He now heads the agency that once turned down his request for help when he wanted to attend a university. They decided he was too disabled and was not employable! As director of the agency that is designed to help handicapped people, Ed Roberts can be a reminder that everyone has potential to be productive.

William Mitchell lost two hands and was burned from his waist to his head when the gas tank of his motorcycle exploded in an accident. He moved to Colorado, learned to ski, drive a car and pilot a plane. About two years later, while flying his plane, he crashed and suffered a broken back. He became a paraplegic. Either of these tragedies would be enough to make many people want to give up. But Mitchell began a new life. He was elected mayor of Crested Butte, Colorado, and toured Washington, D.C. to enlist federal support for environmental issues affecting the town. He is active in his role of mayor and in his own life.

In a syndicated newspaper interview with Cynthia Gorney of the *Washington Post,* Mitchell said, "The way I look at it, before I was paralyzed there were 10,000 things I could do, 10,000 things I was capable of doing. Now there are 9,000. I can dwell on the 1,000 or I can concentrate on the 9,000 I have left."

On a national level, in 1977 President Jimmy Carter picked Max Cleland to head the Veterans Administration. In this position he is the link between government and thirty million American veterans. Max Cleland is a veteran, having served in Vietnam. After losing both legs and an arm when a grenade went off, he spent 18 months in rehabilitation at a Veterans' Hospital. He entered politics and became the youngest member to be elected to the Georgia State Senate, serving two terms from 1970-74. In 1975 he joined the Veterans Affairs Committee of the United States Senate, working on health care issues.

During his first weeks in office Max received a phone call from police who said a veteran had taken a doctor hostage and was holding him as a protest about his not getting adequate care. The veteran told police he would only talk to Max Cleland. Max successfully talked the man into surrendering and promised that he would get proper care and help. Max used his own experience to reach this desperate man, and his own inner strengths served to bridge the gap between the individual needing help and the bureaucracy.

The media are doing more these days to realistically show the plights of the handicapped. One movie I saw recently, *Coming Home* with Jane Fonda and Jon Voight, was filmed in a rehabilitation center for the handicapped. In an article, Jon Voight told how he lived in a wheelchair before playing the role. Movies show their heroes as tall, dark and handsome . . . physically perfect. But the world is not filled with "perfect" people. Movies like *Coming Home* show a side of life that is real and natural.

The Myth About Sex

The movie *Coming Home* was also a love story, depicting an affair between a woman (who came to the hospital to help patients and to fill her time) and a paraplegic. It was an honest portrayal of two people, drawn together and attracted to each other on several levels, including a sexual one. One scene, which was quite explicit, left no doubt that a sexual experience had occurred and that it had been totally successful for both of them. As I came out of the theater, I heard one woman say "I didn't know handicapped people did that!" The myth that handicapped people can't have sexual relations has wide acceptance.

I became aware of sex for paraplegics when Larry was in the spinal cord disability unit where there was sex counseling for patients and families. Since Larry had regained almost total functional abilities by the time he was released, we did not need counseling together, although Larry explained that his sensation level might be somewhat reduced and I might have to be the more active partner. Our biggest block was hesitancy to resume our normal sex life. We were both unsure of how Larry would respond. Given a little time after his homecoming for his adjustment to everything else, our normal closeness provoked the needed desire and our love for each other overcame any uncertainty. In many ways, lovemaking was more impassioned. Larry's regained ability was so miraculous that a new dimension of gratitude was added to sexual pleasure and joy.

Ed Roberts, Director of the California Department of Rehabilitation, is paralyzed from polio. It surprised many people when he married. His wife, Kathy, was formerly his occupational therapist. They have a young son, Lee Brian Roberts. The Roberts are an example of love transcending an apparent problem. Marriage and family are possible for paraplegics. Ed Roberts, in an article written by Linda B. Joffie, said "I want to dispel the notion that disabled people cannot—or should not—have sex."

The subject of sex for the disabled was the conference topic recently in four American cities and Toronto, Canada. With more public exposure through the media and with counseling for the disabled, the sexual myth may soon disappear. If you need counseling, contact your state department of rehabilitation or rehabilitation center.

Family Relationships

Family relationships will be under additional stress with a member disabled. Pressure to any relationship, marriage, parents, friend, will cause change. Some marriages do not survive the strain and end in divorce. Problems develop between parents and children, and between children. Open and honest communication is essential for understanding and as a basis for forming a new life together. Counseling is available. If needed, see your doctor, discharge planner or county social worker.

Some families, on the other hand, seem to come closer in crisis when they have a solid love for each other and a good communication system. All of their strengths seem to be activated by stress. Stories of couples being married after either the bride or groom is disabled are becoming more common.

Attitude—The Biggest Handicap

In other chapters I've discussed the importance of attitude. The people described earlier in this chapter had an attitude that motivated them to a fullness of life. Attitude is always the key to the kind of lives people have. This is not limited to patients; the attitude of families is important to the health and happiness of the entire family. The attitude of medical staff sets the stage for patients and families. And the attitude of the total society lets patients know whether they are accepted as whole people or thought of as "cripples."

The handicapped are becoming a voice for social reform in the community. They have begun to work together in groups to bring about social change. Some changes are happening but more changes are needed. Sometimes the handicapped use sit-ins as a form of protest. Once they persuaded officials in Oakland, California to try to live a day in a wheelchair to help those who make the laws become aware (in some small way) of the problems of the handicapped living in a world made for well people.

About thirty council members were struggling to get through one day in a wheelchair while still performing their duties. The idea was to have one disabled "buddy" for each politician. Not all politicians participated, and some began the day but became frustrated and simply folded up their wheelchairs and resumed normal activities. Some tried, but got up out of the chairs to get a drink of water or push an elevator button when they couldn't function in the chair.

The day may not have been a total success, but two significant things were clearly demonstrated. One, the handicapped are functioning as individuals and in groups, dedicated to living the best life they can while they work for change in the outer world. This exemplifies that some change in attitude has already taken place. And two, that communication is opening up between those who are not physically handicapped and those who are. Open communication is important because we must realize that we are all connected, and that what happens to one of us happens to all of us. Any attempt to understand another human being, who is living in a different set of circumstances, changes your life as well. How can you complain about having to get up and go to work when someone else cannot get up at all or cannot work? How can you criticize another's despair when you react to your own hurts?

These changes in social attitudes are resulting in new opportunities for the "handicapped."

Opportunities

In education admission is easier due to the successful completion of college by pioneer handicapped people like Ed Roberts. Physical facilities are improving in schools and colleges. Ramps are replacing stairs, wider doors and special equipment are being installed. In some states, such as California, funds are guaranteed for the disabled to attend private schools if they cannot be educated in public schools. Education provides new career opportunities previously unavailable to many handicapped people.

Recreational facilities are now being provided in state and federal parks including trails for wheelchairs, convenient parking spaces and adapted restroom facilities. Camps and recreational facilities are now available for the handicapped. Motels are required to have some rooms available for the handicapped to allow travel. Lists of recreational sites, restaurants, even gas stations with accessible facilities are published in some areas.

The National Trust for Historic Preservation initiated a pilot project in 1977 at Cliveden House in Philadelphia to make historic sites accessible to the handicapped. Persons in wheelchairs, walkers, or using canes or crutches can be accommodated by providing ramps instead of steps, and enlarging hallways and doorways. Those with limited sensory perception may use alternative audio-visual equipment to view inaccessible areas. Braille handbooks are also available. A nearby visitor center includes restrooms that conform to the city and state codes for the handicapped. Parking spaces near the main building are reserved for the handicapped. Other centers are also making changes for better accessibility and safety. Gravel paths are being replaced with asphalt, for instance. The National Parks Service conducted a one-day workshop on how to convert existing sites. Staff members of historic sites receive training in assisting handicapped persons. It is estimated that 20% of the total United States population is handicapped. With modifications of historic sites these citizens may soon be able to visit centers previously unavailable to them. Questions about facilities should be directed to the site you wish to visit.

Employment Career opportunities are improving, partly because of educational learning, occupational therapy conducted in rehabilitation centers where patients are re-trained in new professions, private workshops for the handicapped conducted by various organizations, and a media effort initiated to persuade employers to "Hire the Handicapped." The state department of vocational rehabilitation aids the handicapped in training and in finding employment.

Transportation Cars can be equipped with hand controls or other special equipment and vans can be equipped with lifts for wheel chairs. Driver's Education is available through rehabilitation centers or the state department of rehabilitation. Public transportation is being made more available for handicapped people. Some local groups provide special kinds of transportation, also. (Contact your discharge planner or social worker for details.) Airlines provide assistance for the handicapped. You must make reservations in advance, describe your needs to the reservation clerk, try to travel at non-peak dates and times, and use restroom facilities before boarding the plane. When we traveled, Larry had difficulty managing the small airline bathroom facilities even though he walked with a cane. We noted they would not be adequate to accommodate a wheelchair. Airlines do provide wheelchairs at the entrance for passengers and board disabled persons prior to boarding other passengers.

Other community, state and federal buildings are now being adapted and designed with the handicapped in mind. For instance, out of the dreary depths of west Chicago has risen a beautiful new structure through the combined efforts of city architect Jerome R. Butler, Jr. and Stanley Tigerman, Chicago architect. The new building was designed as the Illinois Regional Library for the Blind and Physically Handicapped. The building, dedicated in July, 1978, is esthetically beautiful, but meets all of the needs of the handicapped, including long ramps for wheelchair users, windows at their level of view, easy access to books and card files, use of color for those not totally sightless, counters to accommodate wheelchairs, and with dips in the formica to tell blind people where book stations are located. Braille catalogues are also available. Even a pre-school play area is provided.

It is gratifying to see city government building new facilities remembering the handicapped. Theirs is a life already made difficult and any alleviation of difficulty is a monument to the spirit of those who will better use the facilites.

Hollynn Fuller has been paralyzed since an auto accident. She is married and has two children, both born since the accident. She has helped form a group called EACH, Environmental Access Committee for the Handicapped. They made a film to help communities understand the need for better access to buildings and community facilities.

I want to make a special plea to non-handicapped readers: please do not park in spaces set aside for the handicapped. The reserved spaces are clearly marked and are located near the entrances of schools, stores and other buildings. It is a temptation to pull into such a preferred space—but remember the handicapped need to use those spaces. They are located where one side of the car is unobstructed. The handicapped cannot negotiate getting out of the car in a space with cars on each side nor can they travel great distances to entrances. Handicapped spaces are few in number. If you park in one of the spaces reserved for the handicapped, someone who really needs it may not be able to park. Those who are disabled have enough problems to solve without having the added frustration of not being able to park. Please be considerate.

The telephone company provides many special assistance programs for the handicapped. They develop programs in conjunction with the California State Department of Rehabilitation and the California Public Utilities Commission. Check with your local telephone business office to find out what services are provided in your area.

Organizations for the Handicapped

These vary broadly in different parts of the country. Organizations such as the Society for Crippled Children and Adults, Lung Association, Muscular Dystrophy and Multiple Sclerosis Societies can advise you of other groups and organizations for the handicapped in your area. You can also check with a hospital discharge planner, social worker, department of rehabilitation or rehabilitation center.

The world of the handicapped is improving. Much of the change has been brought about by the vitality of handicapped people. They are providing the inspiration and leadership to bring about further change in both community acceptance and facilities.

Handicapped people overcame obstacles in their lives that would make most of us shudder with horror. The common denominator in all their lives is attitude and spirit. They may not be able to change their circumstances, but they do change their attitude about what constitutes a "good life." Another thing they all seem to have in common is that they have all learned how to give of themselves. Perhaps their own desperate need makes them more understanding of the needs of others, perhaps their handicap (so-called) has taken them out of the hurry-scurry world and given them the blessing of time, perhaps their loss of physical identity has brought them closer emotionally to other people and spiritually to God. Whatever it is, they have something special. It's as if they found the answer to life not in spite of their handicaps, *but through them.*

Chapter X

Care for Children

Home care benefits many groups of people, but those who may benefit most are children. Children associate security with their home and family and have only limited experience away from their own environment. Isolation in a hospital, even for short periods of time, can be traumatic to children. They need nurturing, particularly when they are hurt or ill. Home care provides a familiar setting and an opportunity for parental support, which is essential to the emotional adjustment of children to their illness. The need of children to trust is paramount in their development. Remember, children have an uncanny perception of people's true feelings and the reality of events.

Children's hospitals try to make the institutional experience as pleasant as possible. One of the newest approaches is to have children participate in their own treatment. Doctors and nurses carefully explain treatment procedures. One hospital also uses pre-surgery conferences. The doctor tells the children what to expect, and staff members use puppets to demonstrate techniques such as IV's, shots and anesthesia. The use of the recovery room is explained. Children are then less fearful when they waken after surgery in a strange environment. They respond well to the use of dolls or puppets. Children will talk to puppets when they do not want to communicate with other people.

One nurse who worked in a hospital in Ohio told me how younger children were frightened and often cried when taken from their rooms for X rays or treatment, but they became calm and cheerful when transported in a little red wagon.

Some hospitals have residence facilities for families. Children's Hospital at Stanford University now has a residential home where parents may stay while their children are confined in the hospital for treatment. Dr. M. Harry Jennison, executive director of Children's Hospital at Stanford, was quoted in a recent article by Joseph Torchia, in the *San Francisco Chronicle:* "There is no doubt in my mind that when you have the loving support of a parent nearby, it makes all the difference in the world to a child . . . . Not only does it make for fewer psychological problems, but the child goes through the whole medical process with much less trauma and actually seems to get well faster. Family love—it's the best prescription I can think of."

Children are referred by their doctors to Children's Hospital at Stanford for treatment not available in their area. Families coming from northern California and Nevada now have a home on the Stanford campus during the time their child is being treated at the hospital. The initial $300,000 needed to renovate the property was donated by McDonald's restaurant operation, so the house is called "The Ronald McDonald House." It is the third such facility, the first being in Philadelphia, the second in Chicago. Several others are planned. Parents are charged a minimal fee of $5.00 per day, but the charge is waived if the parents cannot pay. The house is supervised by a group of parents, who can relate to families in crisis. The house helps keep families together during periods of treatment. Parents need help and counseling when their children become ill or are injured. The Ronald McDonald House allows parents to assist each other because of their common problem—seriously ill children. Sometimes it helps just to know you're not the only one facing a problem. Parents can support one another, an excellent form of therapy.

Healthy children, used to a world of sports, games, fun, and friends, find their world suddenly changes when they become seriously ill. They have difficulty understanding what happened to them. Treatment is often trying and painful. Chemotherapy, for instance, may make them sicker than they were before treatment. Older children may have strong preconceived ideas of illness and death. Most children, as a rule, make a remarkable adjustment to their hospitalization and treatment, even though they feel isolated from family and friends.

School is a natural part of a child's life. Hospitalization disrupts a regular academic program and some hospitals have a school for children who require long-term treatment. If a hospital stay is short, the students may be able to return to their own school. Another alternative is a home teaching program. In most cases, families should inform school personnel (teacher, counselor, principal) of the original diagnosis, so the school staff can support the student's continuing education. Realistic academic counseling will be required during treatment.

Occasionally, though, a parent may feel it best to withhold information from the school. One mother felt her son would be in physical danger if other students knew he was in a weakened condition. They lived in a rough neighborhood, and she said there were many fights. Another mother wanted her son to have a "normal" life and felt the students would "pity" him and treat him differently if they knew about his illness.

Students usually welcome the chance to continue their studies, but do not want to be "bugged" to attend classes when they do not feel well. Attendance fluctuates not only in the hospital, but when they return to their own school. They will miss classes when they do not feel well and when they must go to a clinic or hospital for out-patient treatment. If sufficient regular school attendance is not possible, a home teaching program may be planned.

Patients may take advantage of more than one type of teaching assistance, but in all cases, a close relationship with the student's regular school and teacher is needed. They can advise other teachers or tutors and assist students when they return to their own classes. This continuity in education is important, helping the maintenance of a "normal" life for the child.

Schooling in Hospitals

Some children become bored with long-term hospital confinement. They may be concerned about maintaining their academic records. High school students may feel the pressure of keeping up their studies so that they can successfully gain entrance to college. Hospital classes and bedside teaching help children continue their academic work. Parents may want to hire a tutor if the child needs individual instruction.

Students may not attend classes regularly when they do not feel well. Some children are overwhelmed by the gravity of their disease, school work deterioration, depression due to treatment, and loss of social contacts with friends. It may be hard to concentrate on academics when the body is physically ill. At these times, bedside teaching is helpful. If the student does not feel well enough to do regular studies, the teacher may simply read a story.

In spite of the fact that students are plagued with headaches, nausea, infections, and pain, approximately one-half of the students attending hospital classes manage to keep up their normal level of education. Mathematics, foreign languages and science (particularly lab work) are most difficult and may require special tutoring.

Dr. Jordan Wilbur, director of the Children's Cancer Research Center in San Francisco, in a recent article said, "We want them to keep up with their class and we want them to get the message, *we expect you to get well.*" The attitude conveyed may provide more benefit than the actual classes.

There are other differences in the students who attend hospital classes. Some may be hooked up to intravenous bottles, some children are bald from chemotherapy, or have exposed scars from surgery. Besides attending classes, students are taken on picnics and excursions, and indoor recreation is especially planned in the wards. A sign on the classroom wall reads, "Get well. Do as well as you can for as long as you can!"

Home Teaching

The State of California Education Code has a chapter devoted to the education of physically handicapped minors. Regulations and stipulations regarding provision of home teachers are very broadly defined. The home teaching policy is determined by individual school districts. Districts do provide teachers who instruct home-bound students who are physically unable to attend school. A statement from a physician verifying the need of a student for a home teacher is required. Length of absence, qualifying time period, and hours of instruction may vary dramatically between individual school districts and from state to state.

Home teaching can provide a very necessary support to the student and family. Instruction can be individually planned and students can continue regular school work, working at their own pace. These sessions can relieve boredom, lessen anxiety about academic progress, and offer privacy for recovery when treatment affects physical appearance. Home teaching is convenient, and allows the student to stretch existing energy. A positive relationship can also develop with the teacher as an important part of the team effort. Families should check with local school districts to obtain information about teaching assistance.

Return to school may require adjustments. A student who formerly rode a bike to school now may need to be driven. Crutches and wheelchairs necessitate careful planning for stairs, classroom and toilet facilities. Physical changes may precipitate teasing and name-calling. Wigs and hats to hide bald heads (hair loss from chemotherapy) are often an invitation for ridicule. A combination of medication and riding a school bus can cause nausea. Pain can cause students to become irritable, aggressive, or withdrawn. Fatigue may halt or impair physical education activity. Students may need to plan to lie down during lunch periods.

Parents, patients, teachers and school officials need to be aware of potential problems in this area and retain a close relationship with the child. Sometimes friends, when informed, can protect students and "run interference" with other peer group members.

Relationships within the family may suffer when one child is ill. Sick children need more support from parents, sometimes requiring the parents to be at the hospital for long periods or when at home, needing a large amount of their parents' time. Siblings can feel neglected, and parents can feel both physically and emotionally drained during this period. Minor problems with other children can snowball into bigger problems when all family relationships are strained.

Any illness in a family can cause strain. There will be adjustments and restrictions that need to be understood. Openness and sharing of feelings is an opportunity for improved communication. This can be the cohesive ingredient which strengthens the family unit. Counseling is available for all family members when needed, but is more effective if it is ongoing and not used only when events pile up and become unbearable.

The goal, for children as well as adults, is to live as full a life as possible. That includes school, friends, and family. Unless the doctor specifically limits activity for medical reasons, it is therapeutic for children to continue their participation in family and social events.

Sometimes, however, a normal life is difficult for seriously ill children and their families. They require another kind of home care—reluctantly and lovingly given. It needs to be mentioned here because it involves a lot of children and a lot of families. I say "reluctantly given" because some children are kept at home because the families cannot find a place they feel is suitable for institutional care on a long-term basis even when the children need it. They must keep the child at home despite the fact that it is disruptive to other family members, with days full of problems, sleep often interrupted for care, and the family social life and vacations non-existent or difficult.

One case is described in a realistic, troubled, hopeful journal by Josh Greenfeld entitled *A Place For Noah,* about a brain damaged child. The book is a diary of the family's pilgrimage with him. Mr. Greenfeld gives the following statistics: "One out of four children in this country is born with a birth defect; one in eight is serious. One out of every ten suffers from some form of brain damage; one out of thirty-five has mental retardation."

This one statement from the book made me realize that home-care is a big part of the lives of these families and I was touched by his poignant writing of their experiences. This book is must reading for families with children with birth defects. The sharing of the family's low points is bound to have a healing effect on those parents who feel guilty because they become angry, confused, tired, despondent, frustrated, helpless, not living up to the "perfect parent" image. And their highs, their successes, their days when Noah says a new word or actually goes into the bathroom and performs on his own, are bound to provide hope to those parents who look for signs of improvement in their own children.

Josh Greenfeld makes this statement after he and his wife took a short vacation from the pressures of life with Noah and pressures of trying to provide a "normal home life" for their older son, Karl: "But just two days away from the kids and I don't think I could have stood a third day. I bemoan the kids, especially Noah, but I cannot visualize a life without him. Just as I can't visualize a life without Karl. Without Foumi. No matter what I say, no matter what I do, I love Noah more than I can do or say. I want him in my house. I want him in my home. That is his place."

This may be one of the greatest statements in support of home care: "That is his place." It may also be the greatest motivating force for families to do home care. It was for me. Larry wanted to be home. In his home. In our home. And I could not deny him that right.

Children with congenital defects need special care and attention. One of these, an English child whose mother had been given thalidomide during her pregnancy, was Andy, born in 1962 without arms or legs. He had two appendages, mere flippers. Because his family could not cope with the problems surrounding his abnormalities, he spent the first six years of his life in a hospital ward, finally going to live with and be adopted by a middle-aged couple. His touching story and the efforts of his foster parents to give him a normal life are told in *On Giant's Shoulders,* by Marjorie Wallace and Michael Robson. It was published in condensed form in the September, 1978 edition of *Readers Digest.*

Sometimes it is difficult to diagnose whether a child has a physiological illness or a learning disability caused by brain damage. The symptoms are easier to detect than the origin of the symptoms. For instance, a lack of physical coordination could be the result of a neurological illness or a brain dysfunction. Hyperactivity, common in children with learning disabilities, could also be caused by allergy. The first goal of parents who recognize unusual physical or behavioral symptoms should be to seek medical advice from as many doctors as are necessary to correctly diagnose the problem.

Examination might include a test to determine thyroid function, allergy tests, neurological testing (particularly balance and equilibrium), eye and ear evaluations. If the problem is physiological, the doctors will recommend treatment immediately. If it is determined that your child has a learning disability and/or is educationally handicapped, I suggest the following:

1. Get a copy of the diagnosis in writing from the physician.

2. Begin to keep a file of all medical information, doctor's visits, medication given and notes of any telephone conversations you have with medical staff or school personnel. Learning disability children often have medical, academic learning, and behavioral problems. A file of information is essential for monitoring of a child's experience and any changes.

3. If you are not aware of existing laws that benefit handicapped children you can write to your federal congressman or senator, the Department of Health, Education and Welfare, Washington, D.C., your state representatives and/or your local office of public education. Many kinds of educational assistance are available but you must seek them yourself and make application for the appropriate help. You will need all records, including the doctor's diagnosis, for verification of disability.

4. Keep in close touch with your child's teacher. Visit classes when necessary and attend all parent conferences when regularly scheduled. Arrange for special appointments to discuss any questions or problems as they arise. Some public school systems have classes for children with learning disabilities. If not, you may need to search out private schools where programs are offered. Be sure the teachers in charge of classes for the educationally handicapped are certified to teach in this specialized field.

Include copies of all school reports and records in your files at home. If you would like to see your child's file at school, which may include academic or psychological testing results, request a time for someone to show you the records and discuss them with you. Be sure to ask questions if there is anything you don't understand immediately. Parents have a legal right to view their children's records and to request copies of information in the file.

5. Parents with learning disability children have indicated that certain food substances tend to disturb the children's emotional balances. They suggest careful meal planning, and reducing the use of or eliminating sugar, caffeine, artificial food coloring and preservatives (or any other substances recommended by your doctor) from the child's diet. Some soft drinks have both sugar and caffeine, which tend to make children more active and irritable. Read labels carefully before purchasing packaged foods. Preservatives and artificial coloring will be listed.

6. On an emotional level:

(a) consider the child as an individual and do not compare behavior with other children in the family.

(b) have firm rules and routines structured.

(c) keep directions simple and give one at a time.

(d) encourage hobbies that develop individual talent: animal care, cooking, stamp collecting, art, music or any other area of interest.

(e) have one playmate at a time rather than a large group of children which may be over-stimulating.

(f) parents must be understanding, limit television viewing, and supervise selection of programs. Be aware that television viewing may cause anger and irritability. Children with learning disabilities cannot tolerate rapid scene changes, plot variables and fast-paced action.

(g) praise any and all constructive effort or behavior, no matter how seemingly insignificant.

(h) seek professional help and join a parent group for those with learning disability children. Other parents are often the best information resource because they are involved in a similar situation. Local libraries have information and directories of organizations available. Ask your research librarian for assistance in locating these materials. You may also write to:

> The Association for Children with
> Learning Disabilities
> 4156 Library Road
> Pittsburgh, Pennsylvania 15234

Counseling children who have life threatening illnesses is often the subject of conferences that I have attended. After hearing Dr. Gerald Jampolsky, director for the Center for Attitudinal Healing in Tiburon, California, speak at some of them, I became impressed with his concern and obvious affection for the children. I called the center and arranged a visit.

I drove across the Golden Gate Bridge to the small picturesque town of Tiburon, which is located on the bay in Marin County, north of San Francisco. The sun was lowering in the western sky as I drove along the narrow road leading from the freeway to Tiburon. The quaint shops, restaurants, and boats docked along the bay seemed more appropriate for a leisurely tourist visit than a visit to a center where children were counseled for serious illness.

The center was not easy to find. A wooden door between two businesses led down a long alley-like passage to the center, which is very near the boat docking area. I entered a small room that looked like a kitchen. A large comfortable-looking room to my right faced the bay and an office was located to the left. A large paper rainbow hung over the door to one of the rooms. It provided a cheerful effect. If I had a child who was ill, I would welcome such a warm home-like place for counseling.

Steve Ross met with me to discuss the work with children. Steve was articulate and enthusiastic about the center. Our discussion was briefly interrupted by a lady who came in to tell Steve she was taking some of the older children for a cruise on the harbor. After she left, Steve explained that someone had donated the use of a boat. Volunteers and staff accompanied children on the excursion. That answered one of my questions; there was an emphasis on living instead of a morbid anticipation of decline and death.

Dr. Jampolsky's office is nearby. He can see children and their families either at the center or in his office. The children have their own group and help each other by sharing feelings. Groups are also available for parents, who have their own special needs. The staff visits and keeps in touch with children when they are admitted to a hospital for treatment, or are ill at home.

Dr. Jampolsky said the children are very good counselors to each other. The staff is there to support the group, but the great value is in letting the children share with and advise each other. This process not only aids the child receiving help, but has a therapeutic effect on the one giving the advice. Dr. Jampolsky recently appeared on a local television program and one of the children was with him. A friend of mine who saw the program said the child was a scene stealer and was able to discuss illness and the center from personal experience.

Steve showed me a book which the center published. It included drawings done by the children. The sketches touchingly described their fears, their views of illness and treatment, and their capacity to live with their illness.

Dr. Jampolsky asked the children to draw pictures of how they felt about situations in their life, beginning with the experience of going to the hospital. As I was leaving the center, I looked back at Steve. He turned his motorized wheelchair around to bid me goodbye. There was no way you could ignore his own contribution to the work of the center. Steve has muscular dystrophy but evidenced a full life. He doesn't have to verbalize his theory to the children—he lives it. I met another staff member who also displayed warmth and generosity. I walked back to my car feeling grateful that the children, parents, and staff had each other, brought together in what could have been a bleak experience, had it not been for the relationships that developed out of their mutual sharing. Some of the children at the center go into remission and are disease-free for a period of time; some are being maintained through treatment, some suffer deterioration, and some die. But all have someone who cares for them.

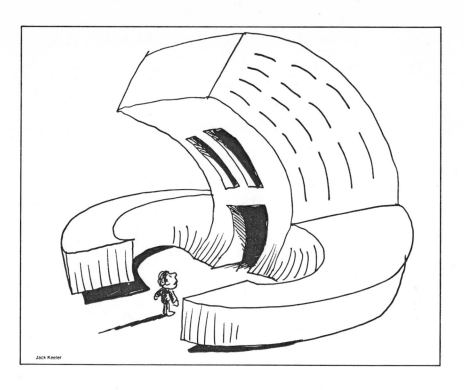

Jack Keeler

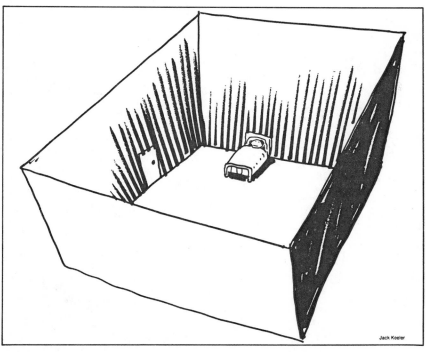

Jack Keeler

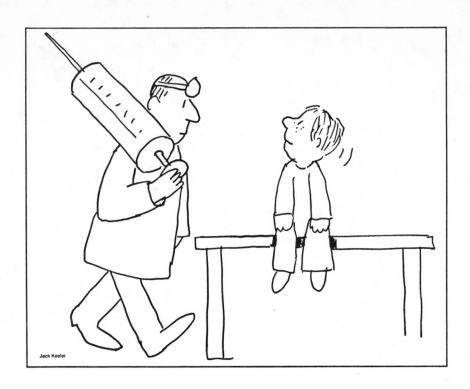

Jack Keeler

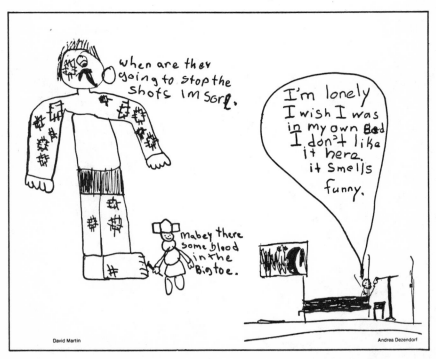

David Martin

Andrea Dezendorf

My meeting with Steve Ross had been brief because the children were due to arrive for a weekly meeting. I still had unanswered questions. The next day I called Dr. Jampolsky's office to arrange an interview with him. I sat by the telephone, calendar and notebook nearby, and waited as the phone rang. I expected a nurse or secretary to answer the phone and I had my "speech" all prepared for her. I was surprised to hear a male voice answer the telephone and even more surprised to know it was Dr. Jampolsky. He was warm and friendly, readily agreeing to the interview.

I traveled back to Tiburon the next week. Dr. Jampolsky's office has windows facing San Francisco, and it is pleasant to sit on the couch and look across the wide expanse of blue bay to the skyline of San Francisco. I set up the tape recorder and we talked for almost an hour. During that time a national television crew came in to prepare for filming, and two children came in to see Dr. Jampolsky prior to the show. Dr. Jampolsky introduced me to them. The girl appeared to be about eight years old, the boy slightly younger. They showed great affection for Dr. Jampolsky and he obviously considered them as friends. Both children had cancer; the boy had leukemia, the girl a brain tumor.

A robot stood on the coffee table, straight and stiff. When the children pushed a button to turn it on, the robot moved mechanically across the table top. Dr. Jampolsky asked the children to explain to me what the robot meant to them. The girl moved to the edge of her chair, picked up the robot and held it out to me. "Okay. You're this robot but you don't want to be this robot. People are bossing you around, telling you how to feel and what you should do and you don't want to be a robot. You are kind of like inside the robot and you step outside this robot and you are you. You know how you want to feel and you can think what you want to think."

Four labels were on the front of the robot. They were "happy," "sad," "angry," and "I'm not a robot." Dr. Jampolsky said, "Now you can also not let people push your buttons."

"I'm not a robot, I am free!" she declared.

"That's right," Dr. Jampolsky said as he smiled at her. "But all of us act as robots sometimes."

"Yes," she nodded, "but we can grow up now."

Adults have told me they feel helpless and dependent when they are ill or handicapped. I could see that children also feel frustrated when they lose control of their lives. The robot provided a way to express those feelings.

Dr. Jampolsky told us his young friend travels a long distance to the center to meet with other children. "Can you tell us about your first visit?" he asked her.

"Well, when I first came, I really didn't understand what this was for. I didn't mix too well with the group. But when I sat down, they explained to me I was here so they could help me. Everybody here has the same problem. It kind of makes you feel at home."

After the children left to go to the center, where a pizza dinner was to be shared by children and staff, Dr. Jampolsky told me that children helping children is a very successful approach. They understand each other's language far better than adults' language. It also gives the children an opportunity to participate rather than be a "robot."

Dr. Jampolsky said the children live at home and go to school. They may go to the hospital for tests or treatment, but the other children in the group continue their relationship by writing, telephoning or visiting the child who is hospitalized.

I asked Dr. Jampolsky how children were treated for pain and if they were given narcotics for pain relief. Dr. Jampolsky talked about pain perception and the use of mental imagery for pain.

As discussed in the chapter on pain, it is impossible to concentrate on more than one thing at a time. If our minds are stuck on pain, the hurt increases. If we move our minds to another area of consciousness with meditation or imagery our awareness of pain decreases. Children can be given narcotics for pain control if needed, but developing pictures in the mind is also effective, he said. Children use imagery to control other physical symptoms such as nausea, which some children have as a result of chemotherapy. Children are receptive to imagery because they have a good imagination process.

My two adult children and my eleven years as a school secretary helped me understand the particular needs of teenagers. Much of their lives is future-oriented. Each academic year is scheduled to prepare students to go to college or the job market. Each year, from grade nine to twelve new dimensions are added to the academic, athletic and social experience. It is a time of more than physical growth from childhood to adulthood—a critical time of changing self- identity. Gaining independence is an important part of this process. Some teenagers, already under enormous pressures, have the added stress of coping with a serious illness. Illness and injury jeopardize the personality development of teenagers. Cancer and other life threatening illnesses put any future plan in peril. Some medical treatments affect their physical appearances like scars from surgery and hair loss from chemotherapy. Injuries may disable them. Lives which should be filled with promise and happiness, which are thought to be destined for the young, become filled with hospitals, medical treatment and emotional uncertainty.

Sharon Winter was seventeen when her cancer was diagnosed. On my visit to the Center for Attitudinal Healing, I saw a letter on the bulletin board which Sharon had written. One sentence said, "Little children taught me how to live through bone marrow tests and spinal taps." I asked Dr. Jampolsky if he thought Sharon would talk with me. He picked up the telephone and called Sharon and asked her if she would agree to an interview. His concern for her and his respect for her privacy reflected their relationship. She agreed to speak with me and a few weeks later I phoned her at home. Sharon was nineteen. Her cancer was diagnosed at Thanksgiving time, about fourteen months before our interview. She described her original diagnosis and treatment, and how these affected her life. She had had chemotherapy and radiation treatment. She described the consultation with her doctor (whom she obviously trusts). He outlined alternatives and planned treatments. He told her of possible side effects:
  1. Nausea often accompanies chemotherapy
  2. She would lose her hair
  3. She might gain weight
  4. She might have problems with her complexion.
All four alter an essential part of a teenager's self-image, and agreeing to accept them was not easy. She said she imagined a metamorphosis of herself into an unlovable, ugly thing. Suddenly, she said she felt the room had no air, that all eyes were watching her. She told the doctor she wanted a two hour leave from the hospital to give her time to sort out her feelings, promising to decide on treatment and return to the hospital. The doctor agreed. Sharon, her parents and her younger brother went to Golden Gate Park, located near the hospital in San Francisco. They watched a young boy and girl playing on some animal statues. In their game, the little girl always won. Finally the boy said, "Well, I won last!" Sharon said she suddenly felt that despite the discovery of her cancer, she was a winner and that she wasn't going to lose everything. Like the boy playing in the park who consistently lost to his sister, and still declared he'd won, she felt a surge of spirit that transcended the situation. Sharon returned to the hospital and began chemotherapy treatment. She described the Christmas holiday season marred by her nausea and discomfort from chemotherapy. This was her senior year in high school, the year expected to be the best year of the four. On New Year's Eve, her friends dropped in, one by one, until over a dozen people were there to help her celebrate the New Year. Sharon said she was very grateful, because she knew they could easily have all gone off to parties. She appreciated their wanting to be with her.

As predicted, Sharon lost her hair and began wearing a wig. During her treatment, her teachers brought books and some brought along colorful scarves she could wear to cover her bald head. She attended school some of the time but had a home tutor the last six months of the school year, and did participate in graduation ceremonies in June.

I asked Sharon about boy friends. The boy friend she had at the time her cancer was diagnosed "took off because he thought I was going to die," Sharon said. Later she dated another young man who totally accepted her despite her changed physical condition, and they developed a good relationship.

Sharon said she now lives in the present. "I can deal with it a lot easier, I can handle it that way," she said. "I have nightmares and get scared when I think of all the 'what if's.'" She thinks attitude is important. "You can be your own worst fault finder. It was a hard way to learn, but I picked up a lot of valuable things during my illness. I don't take things as seriously as I used to. You have to have a sense of humor."

"Don't be afraid to ask question—they might be the right questions," she stated as being essential in medical care. Sharon described the many different ways people reacted to her illness. It was like they no longer saw her as "Sharon—a real person" but instead saw only the cancer. When Sharon joined a group, at the Center for Attitudinal Healing, with children ages seven to seventeen years old, a small boy asked her why she was in the group. She explained she had cancer. The children asked about her treatment. When she told them she was due to have a bone marrow test and spinal tap, and that she was afraid the boy said, "I'll tell you all about that—I've had it done!" He not only explained what the medical staff did during the procedure but he told Sharon how doing imagery during the tests helped him not to be afraid. He said he thought of something else during the time; his toys, eating ice cream, playing with his friends, a family vacation. Sharon said that child taught her how to endure the tests. She did imagery during the procedures, finding things in the room to focus on. She counted flowers in the wallpaper, she thought of anything that would take her mind away from what they were doing to her. She called it "self-hypnosis." The process worked and it was taught to her by small children!

Although she found love and acceptance in her group at the center, in her family and with her close friends, others reacted in different ways. Some became overly protective, some didn't understand, some were afraid to ask questions, some withdrew from her because they couldn't handle her illness. Some assumed she would die and remained silent, while others asked her outright, "Sharon, are you going to die?" Some went on with their lives as if Sharon did not have cancer. Sharon had to learn understanding of their predicament as well as her own. Sharon related having difficulty remembering the painful treatment now. She has overcome the initial shock, the onset of fear and lingering depression. She has regained her own identity within herself—and is no longer preoccupied with being a patient.

At the time of our interview she was attending college classes, had a job, and was spending much of her free time speaking of her experience to groups of patients, medical staff and community groups.

Dr. Jampolsky said their approach at the center is to work closely with the family and the doctor. This team effort is especially important in the final stages of a child's illness. The decision of whether a child should be hospitalized or at home during this time should be made by the family. Dr. Jampolsky observed that more and more families are keeping children at home during this critical time. Families may choose home care because it is less expensive than hospitalization and long-term illnesses can be a financial hardship for families, or they may decide on home care because of the emotional nutrition it provides. Dr. Jampolsky said it seems to work dynamically, positively and practically for families.

The staff and children visit and stay related to a dying child. "People think of the dying process as separation. It is important to have a sense of connection all through a child's last days," Dr. Jampolsky stated.

Dr. Jampolsky and children from the center have made several television appearances, and have been interviewed for magazine and newspaper articles. As a result, Dr. Jampolsky is receiving calls from parents in many parts of the country. They have begun a pen pal program and telephone network. Children of the same age are linked together to help each other. The chain is growing as each one then helps another. Dr. Jampolsky also sends their book *There Is A Rainbow Behind Every Dark Cloud,* and tapes made by the children to assist parents in getting started on their own. Dr. Jampolsky told me there are many things that can be done in the healing process that cost no money but have great value. You don't need a center to begin he pointed out. All it takes is one parent with a sick child connecting with another parent with a sick child. Usually a doctor can give you the names of other parents if you explain that you want to share experiences. You begin the process by helping each other.

Dr. Jampolsky's lectures and his work with the children at the center have a spiritual emphasis. He often used phrases and ideas from the *A Course in Miracles* books which he said "changed his life."

"Children come into this world pure light, pure innocence, pure forgiveness. Then our culture tends to get them involved in a belief structure that tends not to be spiritual. We learn to believe in the finiteness of life. I wouldn't be able to work with the children if I felt the finiteness, that would be too painful for me. I wouldn't experience any joy. We are on a spiritual base and we don't see loss in the same way . . . I think God, and experiencing God is important," Dr. Jampolsky concluded.

The Center for Attitudinal Healing then is a place where attitudes can be changed. These changes take place in the children, medical staff, parents and in volunteers. Changes in attitude do literally change your life. The Center makes no charge for its counseling services. If you are interested in receiving more information, tapes or books you may write to: 19 Main Street, Tiburon, California 94920.

Parents have many professional and community resources available when they need assistance. Doctors supervise all care. Nurses can teach needed skills for home care. Physical, occupational and speech therapists can assist with equipment, mobility training, special therapy and home adaptation. Counseling for children is available. Parents may also need counseling to handle the stress of responsibility and anxiety created from their child's illness. The pressures of acute illness can cause marital problems and the divorce rate is high among parents with severely ill children. It is particularly difficult for parents to accept the fact that they have children who are handicapped.

Dr. Kenneth L. Moses, clinical psychologist, gave a speech at a symposium in February, 1977, in Illinois. Dr. Moses theorizes that parents go through a bereavement process, which he calls "The Mourning Theory," when they discover their children are handicapped. The first stage of the mourning process is denial (I don't believe my child is handicapped or impaired.) Guilt follows, parents feel they are somehow responsible for the handicap, that they caused the impairment. Anger and depression result from guilt feelings. Dr. Moses' lecture is thorough and complete in explaining the mourning process. Parents need to understand and handle their own feelings in order to provide nurturing and support for their children. They must work through denial to seek needed treatment for their children. Fear and depression may cause a parent to be overly protective of children; anger can result in conscious or unconscious rejection of the children. Feelings can also be turned on to a spouse. Since relationships are crucial in dealing with illness and handicaps, parents will need to work through their normal and natural reaction to the shock of having handicapped children before they can be free to objectively help those children. A copy of Dr. Moses' lecture can be obtained by writing to: Julia S. Molloy Education Center, 8701 North

Menard Avenue, Morton Grove, Illinois 60053. There is a small charge. Videotapes of Dr. Moses' lecture, one for parents and one for professionals, are available for counseling purposes.

Siblings may also need counseling to cope with feelings of rejection when parents must necessarily spend considerable time in care and treatment of a brother or sister. Anger and resentment are also common in siblings as is the after feeling of guilt. Most hospitals have chaplains available for parents when children have critical hospital stays. The County Mental Health Associations, Family Service Agencies and non-profit organizations (Multiple Sclerosis, Muscular Dystrophy, American Cancer Society, Easter Seals, etc.) also provide assistance.

A good reference book to keep on hand is *Healing at Home, A Guide to Health Care for Children,* by Mary Howell, M.D., Ph.D.

Chapter XI

Care for the Elderly

Who are the elderly and what choices do they have about how they will live out the last portion of their lives? The dictionary definition of "elderly" is that they are the group of people between middle age and old age. The medical and emotional needs of the elderly are significantly different from other age groups. In this chapter the physiological symptoms and emotional factors are considered. These often determine where and how the elderly live.

It is difficult to determine at what age a person becomes "elderly," because many factors contribute to the assessment of age. It is as much a mistake to deny the aging process as it is to capitulate to the calendar. Some people may live many years and remain mentally alert and physically active; others may show symptoms of aging before the predetermined time considered appropriate for aging to begin. Young people, for instance, can have attitudes that make them appear old, or older persons can have enthusiastic and positive attitudes that make them appear young. Some diseases associated with the elderly occur in younger people. Despite these exceptions, there are symptoms and diseases which are characteristic of the aging process. Rather than "expecting" to develop problems at certain ages, I suggest instead the elderly be aware of their own bodies and physical functioning. Families can be aware of the aging process and prepare themselves to handle physical and emotional problems should they develop.

It would be unrealistic to continually drive a car, piling mile after mile of use on the mechanical parts, and be unaware of the effects of that use. The way a car is driven, the care or lack of care and maintenance, the variety of uses, and how well the car was originally constructed, all contribute to the longevity of the car. As with a car, body structure, usual level of functioning, health care and how bodies have been used or abused have an influence on aging. Normal wear and tear on the physical body is inevitable. It is important to be aware of the possible physical effects of age.

The heart is the most constantly used and vital organ of the body. Since it is the powerhouse of the body and is never totally at rest (it never takes a vacation), it can sometimes merely fail to pump adequately (heart failure), or it can be subject to heart attack.

One problem in the cardio-vascular system is a cardio-vascular accident (CVA), commonly called a "stroke." Another is arteriosclerosis (hardening of the arteries) usually associated with plaque caused by cholesterol deposits in the walls of the arteries, the blood flow to the brain and other parts of the body. This aging of the cardio-vascular system can produce what is commonly called "senility," and is primarily caused by lack of oxygen to the brain. Studies have shown that saturation of the brain with oxygen improved memory, reasoning ability, orientation to time and place and stability. This is done in some parts of the country in large chambers and is called hyperoxygenation therapy.

PHYSICAL CARE

There are different aspects of the care for the elderly due to the changes and biological deterioration consistent with age. With advanced age bones become brittle (a disease process called osteoporosis, depletion of calcium in the bones) which can be caused by poor nutrition, drug therapy, lack of exercise, and/or the genetic predisposition of the individual. If an older person falls, for example, bones break easier, heal more slowly and surgical repair is more difficult and sometimes impossible. Physical therapy may be needed to restore mobility.

Some diseases such as arthritis, neurological diseases such as Parkinson's and multiple sclerosis, emphysema, strokes and cancer are disabling in the elderly. Patients may need both physical and occupational therapy as well as special nursing care and equipment.

Elderly patients often complain about general coldness, particularly cold hands and feet. Even on hot days some will wear sweaters or shawls while sitting in the sun. These symptoms are caused by poor circulation, lack of exercise, or possibly anemia.

Some eye problems can be helped by annual examination and pre-scribed eye glasses but others like glaucoma, cataracts, or detached retinas may need surgery or medical intervention.

Some hearing problems can be helped by hearing aids. Others are neurological in origin and hearing aids will not remedy the loss. Only your physician can tell the difference.

If patients have their own teeth, they should have dental checkups regularly and treatment when needed. If patients have false teeth or dentures, be sure they fit well and are properly maintained.

Two of the areas that signify major changes in the total system are skin and nails. It is vital to maintain healthy skin, to avoid any breakdown, drying, peeling, bruises or wounds. The consistency and texture of the nails can be indicative of a larger problem and should be called to the attention of the doctor.

When you are doing home care for the elderly, it is advisable to be aware of the fact that elderly people need a smaller amount of food than active adults. They may need to eat less and more frequently, rather than their old habit of three heavy meals per day. The larger meal should be served at midday. The gastrointestinal tract can be-come sluggish with age, especially without exercise. Adequate atten-tion to fluid intake and diet can assist the functioning. Heavy intake at an evening meal may cause restlessness, sleep disturbance, and poor elimination. Calories eaten late in the day tend to be stored as fat and excess weight can be a problem.

Most elderly do not exercise enough to burn off extra calories. In some cases, obesity occurs and itself becomes a major health prob-lem. The diet should be well balanced, including the basic four food groups (protein, carbohydrates, fats, and minerals) and if the pa-tient has allergies, you will have to substitute. Unless it is restricted for medical reasons, include some roughage, like bran, whole grain-ed breads, vegetables and fruit. Diet should be appropriate to the in-dividual needs. Vitamin and mineral supplements may be used. Snack foods are popular with the elderly, sometimes because they re-lieve boredom. Some suggestions are fresh fruit, vegetable juices, or liquid drinks made in the blender from a variety of recipes. Protein powder can be mixed with milk (skim milk if you are watching weight) or fruit juice. Try to avoid all snacks made with sugar or those containing extra salt.

Individual preference for alcoholic beverages is a benefit of home care. If patients like a drink before dinner or a small glass of wine and the physician has not indicated disapproval for general health, they may enjoy it. Be alert, however, to habitual or compulsive use of alcohol to relieve boredom. Alcoholism is a recognized major problem in the elderly.

Diet can be used to stimulate normal movement of material through the bowel. Figs as a snack or dessert are helpful. Prunes or prune juice (small glass at breakfast and one at night) may help maintain good function. Good fluid intake of any kind is a must. If problems still persist and are not helped by diet or fluid intake, stool softeners may be indicated. These are sold over the counter in any drug store and the patient may have the kind or flavor they prefer.

Always take into consideration the normal bowel habits of the patient before he became ill. Bowel training usually is done after breakfast but any program is done at the same time every day. Sometimes all that is required is sitting on the commode following the use of a glycerine suppository. If this is not effective, digital stimulation can be used. Daily bowel movements are not necessarily required. If the patient had a regular habit of elimination every other day, this is acceptable and normal for him. It is important to monitor the consistency and color of the stool, however. Find a happy medium between too loose and too solid. If the stool is too loose, eliminate figs and prunes from diet. If too solid, more figs and prunes may be added plus a stool softener.

An impaction (too solidly formed stool which is impossible to force out naturally through the normal musculature) may require manual removal. This entails donning plastic or rubber gloves and using vaseline or other lubricant jelly, reaching in and removing the feces. This requires care to avoid damaging the rectum. Once the impaction is removed normal function should return. Plan carefully so that you always have an adequate supply of lubricant jelly and gloves on hand. Removal of an impaction should occur *before* bathing and linen change.

Knowledge of these conditions is necessary when providing home care but can also be helpful when a family member lives in a community facility. The best prevention of medical crisis is to be alert to change (see chapter on emergencies).

This knowledge can also help the elderly decide in advance how much treatment and what limits they want put on treatment while they are well and alert. Dr. Louis Shattuck Baer has written a book on this subject entitled, *Let The Patient Decide.* Dr. Baer has a family practice and still makes house calls. Because he has practiced for more than thirty years, many of his patients are elderly. He continues to visit them in their home and nursing homes. He is a strong advocate of patients' rights. He believes so strongly in the individual's right to determine treatment and the way they prefer to die, that he wears a Medic Alert identification bracelet. This states, "Positively no resuscitation, no IV, no injection, no intubation," thus setting his own limits on treatment. If the elderly make no choices before illness or injury occurs, there is a possibility they may not be able to decide later. Families will then make the decision "to do everything possible." This decision might be in direct opposition to the patient's wishes. Some might prefer to die naturally rather than to be kept alive permanently by the use of machines. When patients make their own decision they not only ensure that medical staff comply with their wishes, but it relieves the family of the responsibility of making decisions when they are under emotional stress.

SAFETY EQUIPMENT NEEDED

Some injuries, disease or the aging process may cause impairments that necessitate the use of special equipment such as walkers, wheelchairs, canes, hospital bed, etc. (See previous section "Physical Therapy" for details on how to select equipment; you may buy, rent, or borrow equipment and seek the assistance available through physical and occupational therapists).

SEXUALITY IN AGING

Knowledge and research about sexuality in later years has been limited due to some of the misconceptions that sex was not important as people get older. As this myth has been dispelled, more data is available to document the needs and experiences of seniors. Sexual experience for some continues into their eighties.

If the elderly have had an active sex life in earlier years, sexuality can continue as long as it is enjoyed. Like the myth that the handicapped cannot function sexually, there is a myth that sexuality diminishes in the elderly. Fear or anxiety of aging can cause impotence in men, and women who have never enjoyed sex may use their age as an excuse to refrain from intercourse in later years. However, sexuality is a normal part of life and need not be considered impossible or inappropriate due to age. Sexual activity can be continued indefinitely. Sexual fulfillment may be at its peak when both partners are free of the fear of pregnancy. Birth control methods sometimes cause physical and psychological blocks to joyful intercourse. If physical problems arise that interfere with sexual activity, see a physician.

MENTAL AND EMOTIONAL DECLINE

Some personality changes have a physical cause. A tumor on the brain which disrupts function, can sometimes be removed, allowing function to return. Senility, which can produce a general confusion, is caused by decreased oxygen to the brain. When damage thus occurs to the brain, it has no repair technique available. Damage to brain cells or brain stems may be irreversible.

Before labeling any person senile be sure a complete examination has been done and a diagnosis has been made by the physician.

Some behavior may be due to the need to evaluate medications and change dosages. Other "senile" symptoms may be controlled by medications or may be due to some underlying physical or psychological problem which can be controlled. Be sure the symptoms are indeed irreversible.

Some elderly patients, who live in nursing homes or live alone at home, lack stimulation and withdraw into a mental state of exclusion. Withdrawal can be caused by a sense of loss of identity. The aging process, if one is to remain healthy, requires active participation in life and a sense of self-identity and self-worth that matures and changes with years.

Change is inevitable for people of all ages. Men, whose total identity has been job-centered will have to find new images of themselves. Women who identified completely with motherhood will need to find other outlets for their nurturing instincts and will need a change in their self-image—from mothers to women. Elderly persons who hang onto old images—thus tying themselves to the past—miss a great deal of living in the present. It is essential to remain an individual rather than relating totally to a role. Individuals who feel a sense of uniqueness, can remain autonomous and open to change.

The elderly do, however, exist in a social and economic structure of society that gives power in terms of leadership, financial reward and admiration to young and middle-aged people. Even in family structures the elderly diminish in importance, with each succeeding generation taking over more and more leadership in the family. This cycle can be a natural and desirable change, provided the elderly can relinquish responsibility and retain autonomy. The cycle becomes unhealthy when the elderly cannot live in the present, and become obsessed with the past. If they can accept and enjoy the aging process which allows them freedom to gradually grow into the future, they will find fulfillment at this stage of development.

One of the common blocks to enjoying old age is a fear of the future and death. As the years pass friends and family members die, this can trigger fear of one's own death. Added to this fear is a natural sense of loss, fewer relationships and a sense of loneliness. Fear and loneliness combined can result in depression. Everyone experiences loss and bereavement at various times during their lives, but the experience may be more acute for the elderly because they mourn their own loss of living as well as the normal loss of another person. They feel they don't want to die before they've lived—lived and accomplished something. The mourning comes from a sense of unfulfillment and regret over missed opportunities. Some have not accomplished the last task which Erik Erickson describes in "Childhood and Society," that of acceptance of "not being"— physical finiteness.

GAMES OLDER PEOPLE PLAY

"Why didn't you?"—Some elderly people try to retain a feeling of importance by asking, "Why didn't you?" This is not an objective question—it is rather a "parental" questioning. It infers that you were not doing something as well as they think you should have done it. If you get "hooked" into playing this game, you will react in the "child" model and will reply in a defensive or angry way. If you want to avoid playing this game, your reply to the question is from the "adult" position, which means you answer specifically and make it a transferral of information. For instance, "Why didn't you sew the bottom on my dress when you laundered it?" can trigger guilt, and provoke an angry response like, "because I have other things to do!" or provoke an apologetic response—"I should have done it." An objective answer would be "I forgot to do it, but I will do it." or "The button was broken and I need to shop for one that matches."

"Someone did something to me"—This is a "complainer's" strategy to get attention. The game is to find fault with the family, the roommate, the medical staff or friends. It is easy to find "scapegoats." Happiness or unhappiness is not determined by outer events or people's behavior, but is an internal attitude.

"I used to"—can be a way of reliving the past in a constructive way by sharing experiences and knowledge. Older members of the family can use their retirement time in setting forth diaries and information for family genealogies that is invaluable. The negative aspect of "I used to" is the refusal to live in the present and an attempt to regress to "the good old days."

"What ever happened to"—can be another healthy pastime. It shows an alertness and memory for past situations and relationships. When asked as a source of information it can provide a good basis for communication. The negative aspect is when the emphasis is put on illnesses, disasters, tragedies, etc. and the discussion of only these experiences.

Game playing is an attempt to gain attention. It does not matter if it's a temper tantrum and angry outburst, tears, complaining or a "headache." It provides attention. Dr. A. H. Chapman in his book *Put-offs and Come-ons* describes in detail other games older people play.

Any communication, even in the most negative form, is better than no communication at all. Withdrawal is a final form of giving up. As long as patients are still verbalizing, there is spirit remaining. The more spirit, the more opportunity for living, and negative emotions can be transformed into creative, positive ones.

The elderly need to have someone with whom they can talk. The listener must be able to separate legitimate complaints which can be (and should be) corrected, from chronic fault finding.

"My daughter had her bridge group over again on Wednesday and they stayed all afternoon," is general complaining. The daughter (over 60) told me she seldom has guests in her home because her mother complains about it.

or: "My roommate watches nothing but sports on TV and I hate those programs," shows a lack of "give and take" in relationships.

Whether the elderly person lives with the family or in a facility where living quarters are shared, a healthy sharing of space and activities is required.

WHAT ARE HEALTH CARE OPTIONS?

A recent article stated that only 5% of our senior citizens live in institutions. Many of the people who live in nursing facilities do not have significant family ties. Some have physical problems that require full-time nursing care. Sometimes the person makes his or her own decision to live in a skilled nursing facility. Most often, a family member makes the decision. No one likes to break up a family and there is always a certain amount of guilt attached to these difficult decisions. You have the feeling that you have somehow abandoned your relative, no matter how good the facility . . . no matter how much love and care went into the decision. It is sometimes one family member's final decision, though there may be much advice from other family members. *Someone* has to take the responsibility and make the arragements.

I remember when I made the decision for my grandmother. It was the only possible solution. She had lived at home until she was eighty. Her physical condition necessitated full-time care and a restrictive diet. Even though she was eighty, she resented "being put" in with all those "old people." She did not think of herself as "old." She had to adjust to her new home and environment; I had my own adjustment—living with and working through the guilt I felt.

When you have someone living in an institution, some things to remember are:

1. *Visit as often as you reasonably can.* No matter how often you visit or how long you stay, it probably won't entirely satisfy them. They look forward to visits and feel the time passes too quickly when you are there.

2. *Do not tell them specifically when you will visit.* They worry and become upset if something happens that prevents your visiting. The only exception is on special holidays. They like to make advance preparations for parties and enjoy anticipation of a special event.

3. *Be sure to remember them on all holidays,* even insignificant ones. Valentine's Day and the Fourth of July are as important to them as major holidays. Birthdays are especially important to celebrate because they place more significance on their birthdays than any general holiday. Each birthday achieved is a very special occasion, may be their last one, and indicates that the years are important.

4. *Remember them with cards and letters between visits or when you are on vacation.* Getting mail is an important part of daily living and your remembering them reinforces family ties.

5. *Give them gifts and treats.* Special gifts are appropriate for their birthday, Mother's/Father's Day, and Christmas. Since storage space is limited, gifts will need to be selected carefully. New clothing is always a morale booster. Jewelry should be "flashy" but not expensive. Many items become "lost," partly due to the "borrowing" by other patients, many who have lost all sense of personal possession and pick up anything they find; and partly due to theft by low-paid institutional personnel. Loss and theft are a widespread problem in many institutions including schools and acute care hospitals. Other gifts might include cosmetics, stationery, pen, stamps, calendar, photos (mounted or a small album for easy handling), a variety of reading material (some can be obtained in large print if the patient is having sight problems), hobby items (sewing, embroidery, knitting, small games, etc.), sweaters, shawls, slippers, and lap covers. Smaller "treats" can be given on almost every visit. Depending on diet, snacks of fresh fruit, crackers and cheese, fresh vegetable sticks (carrots, celery, etc.) can be given to be eaten with dinner or before bedtime.

6. *Be aware that elderly people need exercise.* Encourage them to walk if possible instead of sit, to have their meals in the dining room and to participate in social events. If they are allowed to go out for walks (even in a wheel chair), the stimulation of the out-of-doors is helpful to their total well-being. Most nursing homes have an exercise program and encourage participation, no matter how limited the patients' function.

7. *The greatest gift*—listening. Patients especially need a responsive ear. It means sorting out the normal attention-getting complaints from the real legitimate matters that need attention. Try to do what you can to remedy those things which are a source of concern and over which you have some control. My grandmother had an intense dislike for fish. She thought she was served fish every meal. Not exactly true, but I did have a talk with the hospital dietician and she marked my grandmother's menu, "NO FISH." On the other hand, my grandmother was raised in the midwest. She believes that the big meal of the day should be served at 5:00 p.m. In the extended care hospital the biggest meal is served at noon, and a light meal at 5:00 p.m. This is because older people need the energy in the middle of the day and because they go to bed so early they do not digest a large meal well in the evening. There was no way I would change that procedure because it was done in her best interest. Over and over I explained this to her when she would mention it to me. I never did change her mind. Her mental eating patterns were strongly set. I tried to be understanding about her feelings but took no direction action as she would have liked.

The need for stimulating conversation gives you a chance for ongoing evaluation of their physical and emotional reactions to their environment.

8. *Develop a good relationship with the medical and other house staff.* They spend more time with your patient than you do. Be courteous and considerate of their efforts but also be firm when your patient needs attention or care. If you have any questions about the care that nursing staff cannot answer, consult your doctor immediately. Also, contact the doctor when a situation requires a change in orders.

9. *Work through your own guilt.* Be consistent and let time help you in the adjustment. If you continue to visit, to listen, to be understanding, to be helpful and when necessary, firm, and mostly loving, the feelings of guilt will diminish. Change is never easy, especially when it involves someone you love.

Some elderly people need assistance in order to stay in their own homes. Check your community resources for this kind of help. The elderly may have children who can help with errands, grocery shopping, meals, and some general home care and maintenance. Others do not have family support and must rely on the community to do things for them. In some areas, there are agencies that deliver meals to the home for a small charge. Information can be obtained from the American Red Cross, county Economic Opportunity Commission (EOC), Senior Nutrition Project, Handy Meals, Little House, area Agency on Aging, Merlin's Residential Dinner Services and Seniors in Action. Costs of meals vary from $1.20 to $3.50. One agency, "Food Advisory Service," delivers groceries when needed. In your area you might begin by calling the American Red Cross and your county agencies. The Family Service Agency is another source of information about this kind of service in your area.

Your telephone directory has listing of agencies that help supply personnel for home care. See listings under Home Care Agencies or Nursing. A Visiting Nursing Association is available in most areas.

When transportation is necessary for visits to the doctor, etc., call your local agencies (heart, lung, cancer, etc.), the Family Service Agencies, or your local transportation firm. There may be a bus company that provides a bus or van to come to your home if you are mobility impaired and have a doctor or agency certify your need. Some areas have special vans with lifts for the handicapped. Also check your telephone listings (in the yellow pages) under Senior Citizen Organizations as another resource.

Day Care Centers are another source of help to both the elderly and their families. These centers operate as an alternative to full-time institutional care, allowing the person to stay at home most of the time but also having the opportunity to go to a center for one day or several days per week. It gives the elderly person a change in environment, needed stimulus and provides a very real service to the family by offering a respite from full-time care.

I recently visited a new Day Care Center in our county. It is operated by a group called the Peninsula Volunteers, a nonprofit organization serving the needs of the elderly. This organization also provides other services: Little House (a center for retired persons), preretirement counseling, scholarships, and apartments for the elderly. On opening day, the community was invited to a reception and tour of the house, a converted four-bedroom residence. Members of the Peninsula Volunteers were on hand to answer questions about the center and its services. Refreshments were cooked in the kitchen and served outside on the large patio. A senior citizen band provided the music. As I toured the house I was impressed by the careful planning that had gone into its preparation. All the rooms were on one level. The large living room, into which one entered the house, was cheerfully decorated in whites, greens and yellows.

Growing plants were prominently displayed in all parts of the house. Three bedrooms were furnished as recreation rooms, where crafts and games could be planned. One room had two stand-up hair dryers and manicure tables. Desks were provided for letter writing and chairs were arranged for sitting and reading. One room was utilized as a bedroom so that the guests could take a nap if they wanted. The kitchen was large and utilitarian. It was a comfortable place, a place I would enthusiastically recommend to those needing this kind of care. I glanced at the menu for the week as I passed through the formal dining room. It equaled any gourmet restaurant!

HOW MUCH CAN BE CHANGED?

The body ages. You can maintain health on a day-to-day basis but you cannot grow younger with the passing of time. You can obtain medical assistance for the treatment of some diseases and injuries, but you cannot replace an amputated leg. You can, however, change your attitude about your physical situation and the aging process in general. A change in attitude can alter the way you live, and heighten your enjoyment of life.

Many elderly begin new lives and find fulfillment in their later years that had eluded them in the earlier part of their lives. Some begin new businesses, formed from their various life experiences. Col. Harlan Sanders did not begin his famous Kentucky Fried Chicken enterprise until after he was past retirement age. He had not been a success in business previously but used his knowledge about chicken dinners to begin a restaurant. Grandma Moses did not become a successful painter until she was considered "aged." Octogenarian George Burns continues making appearances, as does Bob Hope, who is well past sixty-five, the "normal retirement age."

Gloria Swanson, eighty-year-old actress, is quoted as saying "I see no reason why age should be treated as a disease!" A few years ago two senior women joined an over 50 club and began jogging as a hobby. They have competed in many running events and now plan to run a fifty mile distance. Hulda Crooks took up mountain climbing at age sixty-six. She has now climbed Mt. Whitney, the highest peak in California, seventeen times. She also backpacked the 212 mile John Muir trail and began jogging at age seventy. She set a world standard record in the Senior Olympics for ages eighty to eighty-five; she is now eighty-two.

Alberta Hunter left a long career as a jazz singer and worked as a hospital surgical scrub nurse in a hospital in New York for twenty- three years. (The death of her mother led her to become a licensed practical nurse.) At age seventy, when she reached the hospital's mandatory retirement age, she again began making singing appearances. She says she was actually eighty-two at the time she left the hospital!

Retirement can provide the time to pursue interests that the elderly could not enjoy when they worked and raised families. With regained attitudes of childlike wonder, anticipation and inquisitiveness, every day can be full.

The elderly have much to give us. Some volunteer their time and affection in hospitals caring for sick children. Some belong to a group called "Foster Grandparents," a federally sponsored program for children without grandparents. Others belong to senior groups influencing legislation and promoting social concerns, like the "Gray Panthers." "Over 50" clubs and recreation centers are available in most areas where senior citizens can socialize and pursue hobbies. Many volunteer in churches and other organizational work.

Our experiences with the older generation can help us prepare for and grow into our own aging process.

Chapter XII

Terminal Disease

Many illnesses cause death but cancer is most often linked with the "terminal" label. We do not say "terminal heart attack" even though we know heart disease is the number one killer. We do not say "terminal stroke" although strokes can be fatal.

Cancer carries the psychological burden of being known as a hopeless disease, terminating in death. The secondary psychological stigma of cancer is that it causes a slow, painful, disfiguring death. Even worse than the fear of death is the fear of a long-suffering illness.

The word "cancer" strikes fear into the hearts of patients. Doctors use the word "malignancy" when they advise patients of their diagnosis. But patients instantly translate this to "Oh my God, he's telling me I have cancer!" The word and feeling associations are already well-formed and are triggered into consciousness by the doctor's words. Just how widespread the fear of cancer is was illustrated in a recent Gallup poll which asked: "What is the worst thing that can happen to you?" Afflictions listed were: arthritis, polio, loss of limb, tuberculosis, blindness, deafness, heart disease and cancer. Of the people polled, 58% said cancer, 21% named blindness, and 10% picked heart disease. The other five afflictions shared in the remaining percentage. The basic concept creating this fear is: cancer is hopeless and all cancer patients die.

The truth is: cancer is not a hopeless disease; all patients do not die as a result of the malignancy; many cancers do not produce pain; many malignancies are treatable.

The first step in reversing the myth of cancer is to realistically look at the whole life-death process. *Life is terminal.* Every single living organism has a life expectancy—a beginning and an ending. Human beings are no exception. The physical body will die—somewhere along the life journey or ended by the aging process.

This knowledge may seem depressing; however, the depression is caused by a lack of awareness of the coexistence of life *and* death. Our culture centers on life, almost to the total exclusion of death. Other cultures have a familiarity with death and some even give death a more significant role than life. Only when people can accept their own mortality as a natural state of being can they keep all disease, including cancer, in a realistic perspective.

The second step of reversing the myth of cancer is to become knowledgeable about the disease. Misinformation or lack of information can cause needless anxiety.

Recent figures from the American Cancer Institute indicate that in the 1930s only one patient in five survived cancer; today one in three survives. Two million Americans have already been cured and 333,000 more have been treated and are looking forward to the time they can join those ranks when they qualify with a full five-year span without symptoms. Each year these numbers are growing.

The facts prove that not all diagnosed patients die of cancer. It is helpful to be knowledgeable about health and illness, living and dying, before a crisis occurs. This knowledge is not just intellectual information, but an emotional and spiritual maturity as well. Most people, however, begin with crisis and evolve afterwards.

I have known many cancer patients. My father died of lung cancer in the late 1950s. Larry's illness brought us into contact with a variety of patients. Many shared their experiences with me. They all agreed that the most traumatic event of their illness was the shock of finding out they had cancer.

One woman told me she heard absolutely nothing the doctor said after the word "malignancy." She later called the doctor to find out what he advised! Another woman said "malignancy" did not bother her, but the doctor added "widespread," and "you may have three to six months to live." She didn't even remember driving home.

Another woman told me she thought she reacted well in the doctor's office but fainted in the reception room. One man related how he left the doctor's office, went to a bar and stayed drunk for a whole weekend. Another man went back to his office immediately after hearing the diagnosis but had no recollection of working that day.

These are examples of patients absorbing the shock of a diagnosis even though most doctors try to break the news gently, and with concern for their patients. Doctors do not enjoy being the messenger of bad news and most try to communicate this carefully. I don't believe any doctor deliberately sets out to shock patients. Some may have difficulty in communicating, which is interpreted by the patients as coldness. Even with the best communication, the reality of having cancer will shock patients.

The discovery and diagnosis of the disease requires that decisions be made about treatment. These decisions are critical and need careful consideration. *No decision* should be made at the time of diagnosis when patients are in shock. The doctor may outline possible treatment options but the decision for treatment must be made by the patient and his or her family. Questions will need answering, time for a second opinion may be required, side effects may be a consideration, and the patient may want to inform or seek advice from other family members. Personal matters may need to be arranged prior to surgery. Time off from work may be a consideration in chemotherapy and radiation treatments as well as surgery. Consultations with surgeons, chemotherapists and radiologists may also be necessary prior to the onset of treatment.

Ordinarily, cancer patients may receive extended treatment before their illnesses progress to the point at which they are considered "terminal," but patients sometimes receive both the diagnosis of cancer and the "terminal" diagnosis at the same time. Cancer, detected early, has the best chance for successful treatment.

It is vitally important that every person know the seven warning signals of cancer. Sometimes the cancer is present long before symptoms appear. You should be aware of any unusual change in your body. Seemingly insignificant symptoms like weight loss, lack of appetite, prolonged tiredness, and inability to sleep can be indications that the body is reacting in a manner not normal for you. These first signs do not necessarily indicate the presence of cancer, but overlooked, and untreated, can affect the normal functioning of the body and the body's immune system. It is far better to treat the first stages of abnormality than to ignore the body's messages and leave it wide open for further malfunctioning.

Other symptoms are more serious and demand immediate attention.

The seven danger signals of cancer are:

(From the American Cancer Society's public education booklet)
1. Change in bowel or bladder habits

2. A sore that does not heal
3. Unusual bleeding or discharge
4. Thickening or lump in breast or elsewhere
5. Indigestion or difficulty in swallowing
6. Obvious change in wart or mole
7. Nagging cough or hoarseness.
If you have a warning symptom, see your doctor immediately.

The American Cancer Society prints this booklet with the seven warning symptoms as a public service. If you would like a copy, contact your local American Cancer Society office or write to the national headquarters: 219 East 42nd Street, New York, NY 10017.

I had heard or read these symptoms, but like most people, a lot of information was stored in my head. A time came when this stored information was of vital importance.

Larry was energetic and always involved in some kind of exercise. He first did all the Air Force exercises until he reached the top plateau and it was no longer a challenge. He then began doing yoga and finally progressed into jogging. He started running short distances and finally built up his stamina until he ran six miles per day. I used to go and sit and watch him run around and around the track at a local high school. I intermittently tried some of the exercises and running but never really liked anything that was physically strenuous. Even as a child I was a reluctant physical education student (I only did what was required of me and never volunteered for athletic pursuits.) I found the smell of gym clothes, shoes and locker rooms repulsive, and always hoped there would be some way I could get out of participating. I remained healthy all during my school years and couldn't even find an excuse to get out of P.E. by becoming ill. Larry accepted my inertness and my only participation in his athletic hobby was as an active spectator.

Larry had been on a ministerial trip to visit prisons in the Seattle, Washington area. It was in early January, 1972. His return home was delayed two days because of an unusual snow storm in Seattle which closed the airport. He called to ask me to contact his office and have them reschedule all of his appointments to later in the week. He returned home, happy to be back in the Bay Area, and free of the winter elements.

The night he returned from Seattle he went to the hills of Belmont for his "run." When he returned and we were relaxing in front of the fireplace, he reviewed his schedule for the next day, which was considerably more crowded than usual because of his delay in Seattle.

The next morning began like any other morning. Larry went in to shower and I went into the kitchen to prepare breakfast. The coffee was perking loudly and the smell of bacon rose from the skillet as Larry walked into the kitchen. "I can't eat," he said. I thought "What do you mean you can't eat," partly out of puzzlement at the abrupt change in plan and partly in frustration at having food cooking on the stove that wouldn't be eaten. But as I turned and looked at his face I knew something was wrong. "What's the matter," I said.

"I have blood in my urine!" Larry told me.

The flashing red lights went off in my head . . . one of the seven danger signs of cancer! I hoped that it was only a kidney stone or something less serious, but I did know at that moment that one of the possibilities was cancer. "Let me call the doctor while you get dressed," I said.

Our family doctor rose early. He was a wise, warm, loving person and I knew I could call him at home and he would know what to do. The calmness in his voice was soothing and reassuring. I explained the symptom. No, Larry had not had any previous pain or other symptom. I also explained the busy schedule Larry had for the day. He quietly suggested that Larry stop by the emergency room of a local hospital for tests on his way to work. It was still early, I thought, and Larry could still get to work on time if the tests didn't take too long. Larry drove himself to the hospital and I went off to work. He called me later that morning and said that the first tests were not conclusive and they wanted to do more testing. He was admitting himself to the hospital for a day or two.

Immediately after work I went to the hospital, Larry told me all about the tests and shortly after I arrived, a doctor came into the room. He also had a calm, relaxed, confident manner and I liked him instantly. He explained that he was a urologist and that our doctor had asked him to order and evaluate the tests. Although his manner was reassuring, his news was not. He was sure that the X rays and tests indicated a tumor in the right kidney and he was also sure it was malignant. He asked permission to run tests on other organs of the body to determine if they showed signs of malignancy. Of course, we agreed. We spent two long days together at the hospital waiting for all the results. No other tumors were evident.

Larry and I discussed the situation. Although the urologist assured us that Larry's body would function well with only one kidney, we considered the removal of an organ important enough to necessitate getting a second opinion. We asked the urologist if he would object to this. He totally agreed and helped make arrangements for another urologist whom we chose to review the tests and X rays. This was done immediately since surgery was recommended at the earliest possible time.

The second opinion confirmed the original diagnosis and recommendation for surgery.

Larry had heard that some cancers spread to other parts of the body during or after surgery, and discussed this with the doctor. The doctor pointed out the advantages of removing the cancer while it was isolated in one organ and the risks of metastasis (growth in another area) if the tumor was not removed. Larry decided to have the surgery. We were grateful only one kidney was affected and that it and the tumor were removable.

It was fortunate that we knew the seven danger signals of cancer and that we sought immediate treatment. We could have put off going to the hospital "because Larry had a busy schedule."

It is easy to get priorities confused. We live in a busy world and we are all tied to a calendar of events. We don't like having our routines disrupted. I think our experience is typical of many people. We wanted the doctor to give us some instant cure, some pill, some test, some medicine, some advice, *something, anything*—that would allow us to go on with our lives with as little time lost as possible. "I can't be sick—I have an important appointment!" How often do doctors hear that one. Or "When can I go home?—I have things to do." "When can I go back to work?—Do I really have to lose weight?—Do I have to give up smoking?—Just make me well and let me get back to my life—fast!"

There was no quick easy pill to take on this one. This was our first experience with any serious illness and this hospital stay began a long series of doctors, nurses, treatment and learning about Larry's illness!

How Do Patients Handle a "Terminal" Diagnosis?

The problem begins when doctors apply the label "terminal" to the disease. Just the knowledge that you have a terminal disease has a negative impact. If patients believe they are terminally ill, they may resign themselves to their fate. They give up. Their minds become set on death. This can begin a negative process that may result in the thing they fear the most—dying.

I received a letter from the husband of one of my friends. He wrote, "Everything happened so fast. Mary had cancer. The doctor told her she had three months to live. I brought her home from the hospital. She went to bed, faced the wall and waited. She died two weeks later."

After Larry had had cancer for about two years, a reporter from a local newspaper wrote a story about our family. It was a three-page article with pictures, entitled, "Living on the Edge." It dealt with how we lived with terminal illness.

Many people called us for advice and support after reading the article, but one call I remember more vividly than the others. A woman, who was a member of a local church, called because Larry was a minister and because he had cancer. She had gotten a "death sentence," as she put it, from her doctor at a large medical center nearby. Exploratory surgery revealed a malignant abdominal tumor. Radiation had created ulcerations on the skin. She was told no further surgery or radiation could be done. She came home, put everything in order, wrote her son a note, and had all the sleeping pills she needed to commit suicide. While she was preparing for suicide, a neighbor came by to show her the article about Larry. She said she called because suicide did not really square with her religious beliefs. Larry was one of the founders of the Suicide Prevention Bureau in our county, and served on the Board of Directors, and I was familiar with this kind of call. Larry was not home and I realized her need to talk to someone. I listened carefully as she explained she was an older woman, afraid of suffering and pain, but not of dying. She had decided that since she was going to die, she didn't want to die slowly. She wanted to speed up the process.

Maybe, I suggested, she could wait for awhile since she was not in immediate pain. I asked if she had thought of the possibility of taking any kind of experimental treatment. She hadn't, so I suggested that she check into some other options.

She called from time to time after that. I got a note from her the following Christmas. She had gone to a foreign country, had treatment, and was feeling well. She moved to the east coast to be near her son for whatever remaining time she might have. I don't know if she is still alive, but I do know she lived that year, and she enjoyed it.

Others are not so fortunate. Not long ago I read a newspaper account of a couple in their sixties. They were told the husband had cancer and was considered terminal. They came home, talked it over, and decided that since they had lived all of their lives together, they didn't want him to die first leaving her alone. It was all there in the note that relatives found.

According to Ms. Charlotte Ross, executive director of the Suicide Prevention and Crisis Center of San Mateo County, California, a large number of people consider suicide as a solution to long-term suffering. I asked her if they receive calls from people who are terminally ill or in pain—patients who have given up and contemplate suicide.

"Yes," she replied, "we get calls from people who are ill and from people who are in pain. Such people frequently want to know why they should go on and tolerate this. This really isn't a question seeking a reply from us. It's more a question they are asking themselves. We try to help people understand that they are in charge, it's their decision and not someone else's. They're free to make the decision.

"We find that most people will choose to live and can tolerate a lot more when they know it isn't a matter of being forced to endure.

The panic that we hear more often is a result of the fear that they would be subjected to a situation where they are not or could not remain in control, to be put in a hospital and hooked up to a machine. They must know that they are free to give up. In my experience most people in this situation do not contemplate suicide to put an end to living, but only as a means to end or control the process of dying."

Typical of others throughout the country, the Suicide Prevention and Crisis Center here has a twenty-four hour telephone service with a paid professional staff, paraprofessionals trained in this field, and trained volunteers. Training is offered in "befriending" rather than therapy. The therapeutic effect comes from a "helping friendship."

The telephone allows the caller anonymity, Ms. Ross explained. Fears, anger, doubts can all be honestly expressed in a safe situation. Callers have total control of the situation; they can hang up at any time. If trust is developed between the caller and the staff member, it may be possible to get the person to come into the office for further conversations. Family members also call to ask how they can help someone who exhibits suicidal behavior.

There is a national organization of autonomous suicide prevention agencies. California has the most groups but there are groups throughout the United States and other parts of the world.

Suicide prevention workers can also refer callers to other agencies for specialized help. If alcoholism, child abuse, rape, high-risk suicides (those who have attempted suicide before), bereavement, or some other specific crisis is involved, several agencies can work together.

The Suicide Prevention and Crisis Center has speakers, films and brochures available. You can obtain information by writing or calling your local agency. There usually is no charge for counseling or service.

Larry and I were fortunate to have a strong faith and a love of living. The pronouncement that his disease was terminal simply made life more precious to us. We valued the time we had together. We tried to live every moment to the fullest. We felt each day was "bonus time."

The Terminal Label: Fact or Opinion

Many patients ask their doctors, "How long do I have?" They have a right to ask and they have a right to have the doctor's opinion. This is one opinion. Patients may want another opinion. They need always to be aware that, no matter how educated and professional that opinion is, no human being can accurately predict the time of another's demise.

One day while Larry napped, a friend called me. She explained that she was going to die. I knew of her surgery about a year before, but thought the tumor had been completely removed. "No," she told me, "the tumors have metastasized to the bone." The doctor explained she had six months to a year to live. It was sad enough that a doctor had made this judgment . . . but even sadder that she believed him!

"What makes you think he's right?" I asked. "How could he *possibly know?*" He was giving an *opinion.* She like many patients, accepted the opinion as fact.

We talked many times. After she got over that original stumbling block— that of giving up—she began to get information on her disease. She began to find out what could be done to *treat* her condition (indicating a positive approach), and she began to look at her life in a different way.

Three years have passed. She appears to be doing well. She and her husband have taken trips to Europe, Hawaii and Mexico. She has become a grandmother and spends considerable time with her three grandsons. She is beautiful, happy and smiling. She has learned to live with her disease, and is living and enjoying each day.

A friend of my mother's had surgery and her husband was given the diagnosis. "She has cancer everywhere. There was nothing we could do, we simply sewed up the incision." He took the news badly. He left her soon afterwards saying he could not bear to watch her die. Before she became ill, the lady had operated a foster home for retarded babies, so she decided she would return to the one thing that meant something to her. "The babies need me," she said. She could not eat solid food, but she drank liquids and ate popsicles. I saw her recently. She is still caring for retarded babies, still cannot eat solid food, still chews constantly on popsicles, is about fifty pounds thinner than at the time of surgery . . . but it has been *twenty years* since the day the doctors did exploratory surgery and told her the tumors were beyond treatment.

None of Larry's regular doctors ever set a time on his illness. The first hint of a terminal diagnosis came during a search for treatment. We were sent to a medical center to investigate the possibility of new treatment. It was a huge building covering several blocks. We waited in what seemed to be a state of confusion. Patients came and went. They sat in hallways. Doctors discussed patients' cases in the hallway as we sat waiting. The examining rooms were small and had a curtain down the center of the room. Not much privacy here either. We both got the feeling we were being herded like cattle from one place to another. It would have been worth it if some new treatment was available that might benefit Larry, but new treatment was not an option. "Larry is getting the best treatment I can recommend," was the physician's edict.

Larry's original surgery was to remove the right kidney. The tumor had metastasized and Larry now had multiple tumors in both lungs. Additional surgery was not possible. Our investigation of chemotherapy had shown it was ineffective for renal cell carcinoma, so this was not an option either. Radiation was not feasible due to the number of tumors. That left us with immunological treatment, which he was already receiving.

The doctor ended the brief interview, which had taken place in a small lab because he did not have an office, with this advice: "Go home, put your affairs in order, and live hopefully." Somehow the former seemed to conflict with the latter! This was our first indication that a doctor put a limit on treatment available and considered Larry's condition terminal.

We had already put our affairs in order. I had always believed that you should be prepared for death and Larry and I had made out our wills shortly after we were married. One of the advantages of having a terminal illness is that if you have not thought about making a will before, you have the time to do some serious thinking about what you want done with your estate. You need an attorney to draw up a will, and to answer questions about probate. Patients may want to include instructions about funeral arrangements. I was glad that we had done this while we were well, at a time we could be objective. Sometimes it takes a crisis to provide motivation to take care of these arrangements.

The terminal label not only can affect the thinking of patients, but it can affect those around them. All lives are interconnected. Patients must not only be aware of their own feelings, but must be on guard for the negative attitude of those around them.

One cancer victim told me she lost her job shortly after receiving a terminal diagnosis. This was not the reason she was given, of course, but she felt that she was replaced because they did not expect her to live. Her boss had expressed concern that her treatment would require her to take considerable time off. Another insurance company employee returned to work after hospitalization to find his desk cleaned out and a termination of job notice lying on top. He has instituted a job discrimination suit.

Friends and family may have difficulty accepting the "terminal" label. Some people avoid their friends because they cannot deal with the dying process. Others may visit or telephone but feel uncomfortable about how they should act. Some may ask questions out of concern but may sound like they are prying into your life. Some may talk about other people they've known who had cancer. The "eternal optimists" will tell you, "Everything will be OK!" But some, gratefully, are still able to remember you as a person and can share your experience.

There is another detrimental aspect of the "terminal" label. To the extent that the label is accepted by medical staff, aggressive and constructive treatment may be diminished. In Dr. Elisabeth Kubler-Ross' book *On Death and Dying,* she relates the attitude of a nurse who expressed her dismay about the waste of time spent on terminal patients. One nurse friend confided to me that if three patients on a floor put their lights on requesting care, the nurse will go first to the ones they expect to get well and to the terminal patient last. This syndrome has been documented in other books and articles.

A different approach could be taken. Instead of less care, patients considered "terminal" can receive specialized care. In *McCall's* Magazine, 1976, there was an article about Joy Ufema, a nurse in a Pennsylvania hospital who requested she be allowed to work exclusively with the terminally ill. "My responsibility is to see that they die the way they want to." If a family is willing, she encourages patients to go home for their last days. She makes necessary arrangements, talks to the family, and makes house calls.

Some doctors do not feel comfortable when treating terminally ill patients. They somehow feel that if a patient dies, it reflects as a failure on them. Our doctor knew we wanted to be kept informed about Larry's condition, and cooperated in every way possible. While Larry was in the hospital in August, 1976, I read an article in *Journal* magazine about "Medical Secrecy." It polled doctors on how they would react to some situations when it would be necessary to tell patients their conditions. It encouraged patients to ask doctors for facts and to demand them if necessary. Patients have a right to know. If patients choose a doctor they can trust, the relationship will be strong enough for a life and death situation. I knew we were fortunate to have such a doctor, but I also knew if he wasn't, we'd get a new one.

Had that been the case, we would have looked for a doctor we could trust, and that we liked. Dr. Isadore Rosenfeld said it best in an article on choosing a doctor (*San Francisco Chronicle,* July 11, 1978) when he likened choosing a doctor to choosing a spouse, someone you will turn to in sickness, in health, in crisis and in terminal illness. "Imagine," he wrote, "spending your last days on earth looking at the face of someone you dislike, or fear, or in whom you have no confidence. And how awful to have to confide your personal problems to some cold, disinterested fish.''

You also want a doctor with the best medical knowledge of your disease and one who cares about you at all times, particularly if you have what has been diagnosed as a terminal illness.

Larry and I felt strongly about our right to participate in decisions about his treatment. There were always choices. Larry refused to have chemotherapy after we had done an intensive investigation and had consultations with several doctors. This decision was based partly on the lack of success with chemotherapy on renal cell carcinoma, and partly because he was reluctant to endure the possible side effects of the treatment.

He also felt strongly about being kept alive if the only way this could be accomplished was to permanently hook him up to machines. "Machines are fine," he said, "if there is an end to their use. But I do not want to become married to a machine, to live out my life in a hospital.''

It is important that patients participate in decisions about their own treatment or lack of it. Living and dying are personal experiences, and each person should have the right to live and die as he or she wants. If the patient is unable to do this, the family then has the right to make the decision according to the patient's wishes. In this regard I am including *The Patient's Bill of Rights* which is now a California statute. Hospitals post a copy in their building. If you are not familiar with your patient rights, you might consult the following. Copies are available through your local hospital or the American Hospital Association.

BILL OF RIGHTS FOR PATIENTS

The following, in summary form, are the 12 points recommended by the American Hospital Association in its statement:

"1. The patient has the right to considerate and respectful care.

2. The patient has the right to obtain from his physician complete, current information concerning his diagnosis, treatment, and prognosis in terms he can reasonably be expected to understand.

3. The patient has the right to receive from his physician information necessary to give informed consent prior to the start of any procedure and/or treatment.

4. The patient has the right to refuse treatment to the extent permitted by law, and to be informed of the medical consequences of his action.

5. The patient has the right to every consideration of his privacy concerning his own medical care program.

6. The patient has the right to expect that all communications and records pertaining to his care should be treated as confidential.

7. The patient has the right to expect that within its capacity a hospital must make reasonable response to the request of a patient for service.

8. The patient has the right to obtain information as to any relationship of his hospital to other health care and educational institutions insofar as his care is concerned.

9. The patient has the right to be advised if the hospital proposes to engage in or perform human experimentation affecting his care or treatment.

10. The patient has the right to examine and receive an explanation of his bill regardless of source of payment.

11. The patient has the right to expect reasonable continuity of care.

12. The patient has the right to know what hospital rules and regulations apply to his conduct as a patient."

Attitude

I asked one of Larry's doctors if he felt patients' attitudes had any bearing on how they responded to treatment. He told me there was no question in his mind that the ones with the most positive attitude did better physically. Those who gave up and were anxious or depressed were the ones who died the soonest. This was also true in bereavement, he added. Surviving spouses who centered on their loss often developed physical symptoms and some died within a short time.

As mentioned earlier, *Getting Well Again* is the title of a remarkable book written by Dr. O. Carl Simonton, radiation oncologist, and his wife, Stephanie Matthews Simonton, a psychotherapist, with James Creighton.

The Simontons work with cancer patients in a counseling and research center in Fort Worth, Texas, where most of their clients are considered "medically incurable." The book, which I consider "must" reading for cancer patients and their families, gives supportive evidence to the connection between the body, mind and spirit and suggests mental imagery as a tool in healing. Their research proves a definite connection between a positive attitude and the survival rate of patients. Imagery is used to change mental patterns to bring about physiological change and to add a new dimension to the quality of life.

In a previous chapter I wrote about Dr. Hans Selye, who has done extensive research on stress and its effects. In 1973 at the age of sixty-six, Dr. Selye was examined for a lump on his thigh. It was diagnosed as incurable cancer and doctors predicted he had one year to live. "Well, there are two things you can do," Dr. Selye is quoted as saying. "Either sit here and pity yourself for one year and be a man on death row that everyone pities, or do something useful."

Dr. Selye, already a well-known author, began writing his autobiography. He decided to live fully in what time he had. "It's not adding years to your life that counts," he wrote, "it's adding life to your years." Six years later, at age seventy-two, Dr. Selye was considered free of cancer. (From an article in the *National Enquirer,* February 13, 1979)

In his book, *You Can Fight For Your Life,* Dr. Lawrence LeShan has a chapter on stress and susceptibility. His research into the emotional state of his patients and the stress factor led him to provide psychotherapy.

He could not cure cancer, he frankly admits, but he found that he could help his patients to care enough for themselves and what their lives still might be, so they could fight the disease with the entire forces of their new-found emotional strength.

That there was a definite connection between personality and cancer, he had long known; now he had to develop an entirely new approach to therapy in order to help his patients change the emotional situation that prevented them from fighting for their lives. Along with many examples of patient interviews, Dr. LeShan ends his book with guidelines on how to "fight for your life."

Orville Kelly was diagnosed as having lymphocytic lymphoma in 1973, and doctors estimated he had three months to live. At this writing his disease is in regression, well past the three years the doctor predicted.

Kelly decided to live as well as he could for as long as he could. He and his wife broke the news to their children. Then they began to live fully.

Kelly started writing articles about what it was like to have cancer, and he decided to try to help other patients. He invited eighteen cancer patients to meet with him to share their common feelings about their disease. Out of this meeting grew an organization called "Make Today Count." Today this organization has over one hundred chapters throughout the United States. For more information, write Box 303, Burlington, Iowa, 52601.

The following is re-printed from a *Make Today Count* Newsletter, written by Orville Kelly:

How to Live With a Life Threatening Illness

1. Talk about the illness. If it is cancer, call it cancer. You can't make life normal again by trying to hide what is wrong.

2. Accept death as a part of life. It is.

3. Consider each day as another day of life, a gift from God to be enjoyed as fully as possible.

4. Realize that life never is going to be perfect. It wasn't before, and it won't be now.

5. Pray, if you wish. It isn't a sign of weakness; it is your strength.

6. Learn to live with your illness instead of considering yourself dying from it. We are all dying in some manner.

7. Put your friends and relatives at ease youself. If you don't want pity, don't ask for it.

8. Make all practical arrangements for funeral, will, etc., and make certain your family understands them.

9. Set new goals; realize your limitations. Sometimes the simple things of life become the most enjoyable.

10. Discuss your problem with your family, including your children, if possible. After all, your problem is not an individual one.

The Thing That Keeps People Going: Hope

I see no middle ground on this issue. There is either hope or no hope. Even if there is only a "little hope," that little can keep patients going. If there is little hope of a permanent cure, perhaps the hope comes from the possibility of either living longer or living more fully in the time remaining.

I collect information on cancer. Many of the articles describe new treatments, both in this country and in other countries. You may find some hope of a scientific cure, or effective treatment that will prolong life. One recent article entitled, "90% of Cancer will be Successfully Treated or Prevented Within Ten Years," described an international cancer conference attended by leading doctors. They shared information and discussed new treatment techniques.

Another article discusses a new treatment, using radio waves to destroy tumors. Others discuss the use of toxic drugs in new combinations not previously used in chemotherapy. There are numerous articles about the use of vitamin C and other organic materials to stimulate the immune system. Extreme heat can destroy cancer cells. Research continues. There is also the hope that comes from believing in a "miracle."

There are people who have had spontaneous regressions, cures for which there is no scientific explanation.

The significance of all this is simply: don't give up hope.

According to statements made by Dr. Dennis Raziz, Director of the Cancer Institute of Piraeus, Greece, there are possibilities of cures, miraculous if you want to call them that, but cures and regressions that defy medical explanation.

"Cancer victims and their doctors should never give up hope," he said in an article printed by the *National Enquirer* (February 27, 1979). "No matter how serious the disease there is always that last chance of a miracle cure in the medical sense." He went on to exhort doctors to continue to fight for the lives of their patients, even if it appears the end is only a few weeks off, in the hope of that cure or regression.

Hope may be all you have left, but it is a powerful weapon. There are several aspects to hope: there is hope for achieving what you desire. Cancer patients may desire to be cancer-free. The hope is that this *may* happen.

Hope also extends to belief in other people. Patients need total trust and confidence in doctors and medical staff to provide the most effective and aggressive medical treatment. Hope extends to relationships with family and friends. Patients need the emotional support of others.

There is hope in being able to improve the quality of life. And finally, there is hope on a spiritual level—to provide meaning for all events of life, including illness, and when required, dying.

From whatever source, for whatever reason that makes sense to you, hope is the driving force in successfully facing terminal illness.

Chapter XIII

The Final Journey

I admired the beauty while I was human:
Now I am part of the beauty.
I wander in the air, being mostly gas and
water and flow in the ocean;
Touch you and Asia at the same moment, have
a hand in sunrises and the glow of this grass.
I left the light precipitate of ashes to earth
for a love token.

> Robinson Jeffers
> *Descent to the Dead*
> (1931)

Birth and death are personal experiences. We journey alone. Our entry and exit from what we call life are solitary. I first became aware of this when I was pregnant. The conception of the child came about as a result of a sexual union with my husband—a shared event. I had a large family with whom the news was shared. *We* all prepared for the birth of the child. We sewed, fixed up a room, furnished a layette of clothes and other care items; and then we waited. My child was two weeks overdue and everyone watched me as if I were a time bomb that failed to go off on schedule.

When the labor pains finally began, there was great activity and joyous anticipation. My parents and my husband accompanied me to the hospital. We're going to have our baby, I thought. The shock hit when we arrived at the hospital and I was separated from my family. "Come along," the nurse said. I looked at her beckoning me down a long, empty hallway. At that moment I realized that *we* weren't going to have a baby, *I* was going to have a baby. It was my experience, mine alone. I said my goodbyes and followed the nurse down the corridor. I was placed in an isolated, bleak labor room. I was alone, I was in pain and I was terrified.

The birth of a child is one of the most mysterious, joyful events we can experience. But my loneliness, feeling of separation and panic kept me from experiencing the true reality of the birth process.

So it is with dying. Our misconceptions about death, which result in fear, keep us from the beauty and joy of our final transition. Many people fear death. They believe that life has a beginning and that we travel along a linear age line until we hit an end.

The ancient men of the sea believed the earth was flat. It looked flat. Ships going out to the horizon line seemed to disappear. The sailors logically concluded that the ships must have dropped off the edge and fallen into a black abyss. Their belief in this theory instilled such fear that voyagers did not venture far from shore. Eventually, the theory was questioned, and the discovery that the earth was round was made by someone who theorized that you could begin at one point of the circle, travel all around the periphery and end up where you began and was brave enough to try it. This new insight, once proven, opened the door to new exploration of the world. The earth did not change, it was always round. What changed was man's view of the world, his mental attitude.

We may view life as a line, with an end called death, or we can view the life process as a circle that we travel, returning to the place from which we started. Many people question where we're going after death but few ask where we came from or even relate the two. If we see life as a circle—the beginning is the ending, the ending is the beginning.

The goal in medicine is health and the prolongation of life. Technological advances have pushed the life expectancy into the seventieth year. This provides great comfort for those who believe in the linear existence. The line is expected to be longer, with death off in the distant future, to be avoided as long as possible. For those who believe in the circle of life, death is a natural part of the whole and is a return to the place from which we came; a going home.

The concept of death and of how to work with dying patients is changing. Much of this change has been brought about by doctors. Two of the best known are Elisabeth Kubler-Ross and Dr. Raymond A. Moody, Jr. Dr. Kubler-Ross has written a book entitled *On Death and Dying* which explores old attitudes about death and dying, the fear of dying and the five stages of the dying process which she lists as:

1. denial and isolation
2. anger
3. bargaining
4. depression
5. acceptance.

Dr. Raymond Moody's book *Life after Life* is an account of his research into the experiences of people who were diagnosed clinically dead but who came back to life and remembered the events during the time of "death." There are striking similarities in their accounts. They describe an awareness of events which continue after the body itself is dead. This consciousness is described as "complete" or "whole"—and they feel a sense of well-being, peace and joy.

Both Drs. Kubler-Ross and Moody have written about their findings, which of course, were only made possible by the willingness of dying patients to share their experiences. This openness provides great benefit to those in the medical profession and to all of us who will, at some time, follow their path.

One of the benefits of a terminal illness is that patients are aware of the possibility of death. They have time to look at their lives, establish priorities, renew or strengthen relationships, and examine their attitude about death. They also have the right to participate in their own treatment, and their dying. Walter Johnson, chaplain at Peninsula Hospital, Burlingame, California, gave me a copy of "The Dying Person's Bill of Rights." He said the author is unknown.

THE DYING PERSON'S "BILL OF RIGHTS"

I have the right to be treated as a living human being until I die.

I have the right to maintain a sense of hopefulness, however changing its focus may be.

I have the right to be cared for by those who can maintain a sense of hopefulness, however changing this might be.

I have the right to express my feelings and emotions about my approaching death in my own way.

I have the right to participate in decisions concerning my care.

I have the right to expect continuing medical and nursing attention even though "cure" goals must be changed to "comfort" goals.

I have the right not to die alone.

I have the right to be free of pain.

I have the right to have my questions answered honestly.

I have the right not to be deceived.

I have the right to have help from and for my family in accepting my death.

I have the right to die in peace and dignity.

I have the right to retain my individuality and not be judged for my decisions which may be contrary to beliefs of others.

I have the right to discuss and enlarge my religious and/or spiritual experiences, whatever these may mean to others.

I have the right to expect that the sanctity of the human body will be respected after death.

I have the right to be cared for by caring, sensitive, knowledgeable people who will attempt to understand my needs and will be able to gain some satisfaction in helping me face my death.

Even in the last days or weeks of life, patients have choices. They can choose whether they want to spend their final time at home or in a hospital. Home care for the dying utilizes all of the medical, emotional and spiritual suggestions given in earlier chapters. The home offers the greatest freedom to fulfill the person's last requests. Hospitals and skilled care facilities are an option when home care cannot be provided.

Dora, in her late seventies, was housebound with arthritis and a leg ulcer. She spent most of her time in a chair, moving only occasionally on crutches. She had no family and lived alone. Despite recommendations by health personnel, who felt her condition warranted some kind of institutional care,

Dora decided to stay at home. She utilized the visits of delivery men, nurses and friends to assist her by doing things she could not do for herself. She was determined to live and die at home, and she was successful in both.

Some diseases, like strokes, may cause considerable damage requiring long-term, possibly limited rehabilitation. In these cases, institutional care provides a needed service.

For example: A wife and mother of four small children had a stroke which not only paralyzed one side of her body but caused brain dysfunction so severe that her nursing care needs could not be met by her husband, who worked full time. This man has three areas of concern. His children must be cared for, his wife must be cared for and he needed to remain employed in order to support the entire family. The hospital provided the best medical and rehabilitation care for his wife.

Sometimes circumstances prohibit the keeping of a promise made to a loved one. An elderly couple agreed that in the event of a terminal illness, each would care for the other at home. The husband adamantly expressed a desire not to die in a hospital. When he became ill with a viral infection, the doctor suggested hospitalization for a few days until he could recover. The wife admitted her husband to the hospital for treatment. He developed pneumonia, was transferred to intensive care, where he received both intravenous feeding for dehydration and oxygen. He later had blood transfusions. Once hooked up to these three devices, he had lost his option to go home. His condition worsened and he died a few days later. The wife could not keep her promise to him, but she had made the best decision for him on the occasion of each choice.

Families are not to blame when circumstances limit choices and they have made each decision in the best interest of the patients considering each individual circumstance. No one option fits every person or situation. Another approach to care for the dying is gaining recognition, that of hospice care. Although interest in the hospice concept is new, the concept itself is old.

HOSPICE

Hospice is the name originally used to describe a way station for travelers in medieval times. It was a stopping-off place where sick and weary travelers could rest before continuing their journey. Hospices provided a place of transition, a place for rest in peaceful surroundings, and a preparation for saying the final goodbye. In the context of working with the terminally ill, the name is applied to the journey the person is making from birth to death.

The whole concept is centered on providing the best possible care for the "terminal" patient. The emphasis is on good, solid, aggressive medical treatment, combined with emotional and spiritual support when needed. All treatment is given to answer the needs of individual patients and their families.

Some areas have hospice facilities either as a separate entity or as a part of a hospital facility (sometimes called a Palliative Care Unit). The hospice concept is also used to support home care. Hospice groups can provide services for patients and families in either setting.

Families are considered part of the "team." In a hospice facility families may come and go as they want, there are no visiting hours. Families are encouraged to participate in the care of the patient. They may feed the patient or perform other duties if they want to be included in the patient's care. Children are encouraged to visit. Special play areas are designed so the children will be able to spend time with the patient. Often, the patient may also have a pet with him. A relaxed and homelike atmosphere is maintained in combination with good medical treatment. Birthday celebrations and other social events are encouraged. Hospices are designed not as a warehouse for the dying but rather as a place for *living*.

Volunteers are also part of the "team." They provide valuable assistance and advice to patient, family and staff. Hospice care begins with pain control and the treatment of physical symptoms such as vomiting, pain, weakness, thirst, dehydration, lack of appetite, constipation, shortness of breath, dry or broken skin, etc. The first goal is to make the patient comfortable. Patients can be depressed due to physical discomfort. If the symptom is brought under control, the depression will be relieved also. Physical symptoms interfere with normal living. A patient who is vomiting will not want visitors. A patient in pain may not feel like making decisions that may need to be made. Oral medication can help the patient become pain-free, awake and alert rather than sedated. When symptoms are alleviated or controlled, patients can then deal more constructively with family concerns, relationships, financial and estate matters, and generally become a part of the life process.

Dying patients have a great deal of anxiety about the families they will leave behind and it is comforting for them to know the hospice team will be available to help families through the bereavement process.

When all treatment possible has been given and death is imminent, the patient, family and hospice team all share the experience. The hospice team provides emotional support for the family after death has occurred, helps with funeral arrangements, attends the funeral, and provides ongoing grief and bereavement counseling.

It is estimated that approximately two million families are now actively dealing with death. One of the aims of hospice is to make the experience as constructive as possible. Death is a normal life experience, one that we will all at one time experience, and share with others many times during our lifetime.

The first hospice was developed at St. Christopher's in England (England now has about twenty-five hospices). St. Christopher's served as a model for a hospice in Montreal, Canada. These two in turn served as models for the first hospices in the United States.

Helaine Dawson is an instructor in psychosocial care of the dying and bereaved at Merritt College in Oakland, California, and in gerontology at Vista College in Berkeley, California; a consultant in multi-cultural communication; lecturer and author of the award winning book *On the Outskirts of Hope,* (McGraw-Hill), 1968, on educating youth from poverty areas; member of the Association for Humanistic Psychology; Foundation of Thanatology, New York; and the Western Gerontological Society.

Helaine and I share an interest in hospices. I had hoped to be able to visit St. Christopher's before writing this book. I was not able to make the trip but Helaine consented to write the following article about St. Christopher's. It describes the hospice concept and its application:

ST. CHRISTOPHER'S HOSPICE

My recent visit to St. Christopher's Hospice in South London was a unique experience which filled me with awe, admiration and enlightenment. What impressed me most was the loving attention and sharing of caring for dying patients and their families by every member of staff, including doctors.

Any discussion of the burgeoning hospice movement in the United States would be remiss without acknowledging its debt to St. Christopher's Hospice as a model and source of inspiration and comfort for terminally ill patients and their families.

Doctor Cicely Saunders, its founder, would be the first to minimize her contributions to the field of thanatology and object to pioneer being used to designate her and St. Christopher's Hospice. The real pioneers, she insists, are St. Joseph's in Hackney, St. Luke's in Bayswater, the Hostel of God and the first Marie Curie Home in London. It was while working with dying patients at St. Joseph's that she saw the need for setting up a hospice where she could incorporate changes she found necessary to meet the total complex needs of patients and their families. Her multi-disciplinary background proved to be an asset. Trained as a nurse at the Nightingale School, St. Thomas Hospital, during World War II she served in that capacity for the duration, obtaining a degree later in philosophy, politics and economics and a diploma in Public Administration at Oxford. Her next assignment in 1947 was assistant almoner (medical social worker) at St. Thomas. It was here her interest in the problems of terminal illness was pursued. In 1951 she decided that such work demanded more medical training which she received at St. Thomas. Following this, she completed a three-year Fellowship in the Department of Pharmacology at St. Mary's Medical School. It was here that she conducted research into analgesics and other drugs now used at St. Christopher's to relieve pain and other symptoms of the terminally ill.

With an initial contribution of approximately $1,000 from a patient at St. Thomas and with the cooperation of other patients and similarly interested persons but still with no site or building, St. Christopher's Hospice was conceived. In 1967 as a result of more intensive work, patience, fortitude, more generosity and with the assurance of two-thirds of their annual budget from the National Health Service, St. Christopher's Hospice became a reality.

At the time of my visit there was a ward block for fifty-four patients in process of being increased to sixty-two. This number does not take into consideration accommodations for seventeen elderly people, not patients, but with no families nor lodgings, who were the original residents when this site was purchased. Instead of being evicted they were welcomed, have access to the dining room for all meals and nursing care when needed. In addition there is an out-patient building housing the home-care unit, a special operation for research into bereavement, a laboratory for continuing research into drugs and a large, separate unit for training hospice personnel.

To encourage accessibility for family and friends, prospective patients must reside within a six-mile radius of the hospice. The general practitioner initiates the admission process after conferences with the patient and family and becomes the key medical liaison with the hospice team. The usual length of stay is twelve days. During this period, however, the patient may return home if he wishes, where he will continue to receive quality home care. A home-care team of doctor, nurse and health service sister (medical social worker) instructs the family in controlling pain and keeping the patient free from distressful symptoms.

If an emergency arises any hour of the day or night, it is handled immediately. Everything is done to heal. According to Doctor Saunders, healing in terminal illness "does not mean assisting someone to get better, but to heal by easing the pains of dying or allowing someone to die when the time has come." To fulfill this objective even further, both patient and family are assured that there will always be a bed ready whenever the patient decides to return to the hospice.

The head nurse, the matron, instead of waiting for the patient to be brought upstairs, comes down to meet him/her. A bed, not a gurney, assigned to the patient for the duration with his name affixed to the headboard in bold type, is wheeled down and he is gently lifted into it. For his comfort the bed has been preheated and the hot water bag remains with him. Since nursing care is on a one-to-one basis, he will meet his nurse as soon as he enters the room of his choice, either a ward room with four beds or a private room. Patients with facial lesions or for any other reasons may require a private room. All rooms are spacious, light and airy. In the four-bed wards, two beds face each other with no curtains surrounding them. We shall understand why later.

Everything is done to make the patient feel at home. If he wants his plants, family pictures, dolls, pet birds, vases or anything that will help simulate a homelike environment, he is welcome to have them. Clutter is never a problem nor a restriction. A hospice is not a hospital with strict observance of rules and regulations curtailing visiting hours and restricting visits from young children. Family and friends and children are free to visit and remain around the clock. There are no parking meters at the bedside.

The majority of patients fall within the middle and upper age groups. Occasionally teenagers are admitted. In this case a private room is usually arranged so that the young person can have complete privacy. The youth is encouraged to entertain friends with rock and roll records on the stereo, sit on cushions piled helter-skelter on the floor, dance and enjoy every moment together. The patient is encouraged to live as fully as possible until he dies. An occupational therapist is on hand for those whose creative energies need an outlet. No wonder Steve, eighteen years old and dying of bone cancer, met his death so peacefully.

In the early days of the hospice, patients suffering from multiple sclerosis were also accepted. Now it is restricted to those with cancer. Why? According to the doctor who spoke to us, the multiple sclerotic patient requires different kinds of attention which seem to conflict with those given to cancer patients. In the latter illness the aim is to encourage the patient to be active and ambulatory, to feed himself, wash himself and assume greater responsibility for his care, whereas the patient with multiple sclerosis of necessity has to become more dependent on others to satisfy his basic needs. When cancer patients observed these differences and anger was aroused, the admission policy was changed.

Any distressful symptoms the patient may have on arrival are brought under control immediately with relief from pain receiving priority. The amount and combination of drugs discussed with the patient's general practitioner and hospice doctors are administered every four hours routinely, a cardinal rule established by Doctor Saunders for the control of pain. The nurse in her hospice training is instructed not to wait until the patient asks for relief. Doctor Saunders has learned that patients may wait too long and suffer needlessly or ask too soon and become dependent. Addiction hardly ever occurs but if a patient is admitted with this problem, it is soon brought under control by giving a proper dosage on a regular basis. When the patient is assured of prompt relief and not anticipating pain, his fears and tension are naturally reduced. This calls for nurse's constant observation and evaluation. Hospice doctors depend a great deal on the nurse's discretion in giving the drugs prescribed, knowing full well that if any emergency arises they will be notified. The amount of drugs each patient receives varies with the individual's condition and reactions and may be increased or reduced as intensity of pain warrants.

Often, however, Doctor Saunders has discovered the patient's pain may be more psychic than physical, and with loving care having a placebo effect, lower dosages can then be prescribed. It is only natural, too, that as the patient becomes more accustomed to the hospice environment, distress is relieved and only local heat may be required to ease pain even when severe.

For example, Mrs. W., fifty-four years old, was admitted in the final stages of carcinoma of the cervix which had metastasized to the vulva and combined with a urinary infection, which added greatly to her discomfort. While these symptoms were being managed with heat applications, analgesics and antibiotics Doctor Saunders spent much time with her until she felt comfortable enough to talk about her real fears: guilt over her past sins and therefore cancer as her punishment. Spiritual help seemed necessary and a chaplain was called in. Soon she was able to reach a state of tranquility. Doctors and nurses engaged in the total care of a patient are urged not to wait to call for such help at the last moment, but to consider the clergyman an important member of the hospice team early in the process.

Often patients arrive with intractable vomiting, dehydration, loss of appetite, malnutrition and/or constipation. Each of these symptoms can be brought under control. Constipation is a constant threat to the patient's comfort and therefore palliative means are used immediately to relieve discomfort. For those patients too weak to sit up and whose mouths are dry and lips parched, the nurse gently wipes the patient's mouth with a wet cloth frequently throughout the day. For those with loss of appetite, food the patient prefers is served in small portions frequently during the day until gradually the patient can return to a normal schedule. Since the relationship between patient and nurse is on a one-to-one basis, the patient feels secure and not apprehensive about her rushing off to care for twenty other patients. There is time, therefore, for those patients unable to feed themselves to be spoon fed with loving attention. Everything is done to increase the patient's appetite. The evening meal can be accompanied by a free glass of beer, wine or whiskey if the patient so desires. On pub nights, however, introduced following patients' suggestions, drinks have to be bought for a nominal cost. This is to maintain the patient's ego and dignity. Thursday nights have been so designated. For the men and women no longer ambulatory, their beds are wheeled into the recreation room where a nurse tends the bar and sells the drinks. The doctor described an evening. At first, the nurse-bartender was ill at ease, but as the evening wore on she became much more involved enjoying the festivities as much as the patients. From a quiet, stiff atmosphere, the room later seemed to explode with laughter, conversation and music. It would be difficult to believe that these merrymakers were dying.

There are now activities daily except Mondays covering a variety of interests. When I visited I saw patients sewing, reading, conversing or resting. The same thing was taking place in the wards. When weather permits, beds are wheeled outside to the lawn where a kaleidoscope of colors in the garden abounds. One patient, an elderly man, emaciated and weak, smiled and said, "College students?" I went over to his bed, placed my hand on his shoulder and said, "Thank you for the compliment." He smiled graciously.

A nurse's day is a long one, from nine in the morning to midnight and midnight to nine in the morning. Although the salary is low, there is no dearth of supply nor is there much turnover. Nurses seem to feel privileged to be accepted by St. Christopher's. The important role of the hospice nurse demands a special kind of person with compassion, patience, openness, self-confidence, inner strength, sensitivity, flexibility, ability to listen and to cope with emotional stress and still be a comfort to patient and family. These qualities supplement her technical knowledge. Doctors respect nurses' skills, judgment, observation and suggestions, considering them *partners* rather than *subordinates* in the total care of the terminally ill. They consult with nurses regularly and as often as necessary around the clock. Neither time nor energy are wasted on trivia. Cooperation rather than competition prevails. Nurses are encouraged in their hospice training to become involved with patient and family. Whatever bothers them affects the patient's equilibrium and therefore becomes critical.

Nurses, no matter what institution they come from, wear similar uniforms: longish gray, starched cotton dresses, white cotton aprons, highly starched, and hats all of the same style. I mention this because in the United States each style hat signifies the nurse's school of education.

Not only is there little turnover of nursing staff at St. Christopher's but of other members of staff, too, like cooks and housemen (orderlies). Possibly the following facilities account for this. Staff members are allowed to bring their preschool children with them daily during their working day. Here at the hospice they are cared for, given meals, naps, recreation for what is equivalent to one dollar a day. This astounded me. I saw nine-month-old infants tucked in and sleeping while the active older ones were outside playing on the green with zestful exuberance.

Does a patient at St. Christopher's know he's dying when he arrives? Should he be told? I was amazed to learn from the doctor presiding over the afternoon session that seventy-five percent of the patients appear not to know they are dying. Facial expressions, avoidance of the subject and the patient's own deteriorating physical condition surely must furnish clues contrary to this. A few patients in the closeness that naturally develops between them and nurses may talk about dying without ever mentioning the word in a symbolic manner, revealing how much they really know. "I hope my wife comes today." "I hope I'm still here tomorrow morning." No unrealistic hopes of getting better are expressed. Even if the patient asks the nurse questions about dying, she is instructued not to pursue the topic but to discuss the patient's feelings with the doctor. The policy endorsed by Doctor Saunders has been for doctors not to approach the question head on, but to listen and let the patient be the one to initiate the topic. The hematologist on staff cited an example in her recent experience. She visited a seventy-year-old female patient, dying of cancer of the stomach, who said, "Doctor, I'm getting weaker and weaker and more tired each day. Am I dying?" There was a pause, the doctor held her hand soothingly and asked, "How tired are you now? How weak do you feel?" They looked at each other and there was instant communication.

The influence of doctors like Doctor Elisabeth Kubler-Ross, who advocates direct confrontation with the patient on his dying, is causing Doctor Saunders to change her policy on an individual basis. For example, Mrs. H., forty-four years old, a patient for two weeks at St. Christopher's, dying of uterine cancer, demanded to know if she were dying. As Doctor Saunder's visit progressed and Mrs. H. became more restless and persistent saying, "Doctor, I've asked again and again what's happening to me but no one would tell me the truth. I think it's wrong if you want to know." She was told the truth. This she accepted with gratitude because she could now plan to finish unfinished business with her husband and family.

Whether doctors are to be direct or not depends on the patient's psychological and emotional development. The doctor has to be careful and respect the patient's choice. To discuss the question of dying with the patient prematurely may create internal havoc and even destroy any small semblance of hope. Doctor Saunders believes that "hope grows as we try to meet the challenges that face us as honestly as we can—in dying as well as in living. It springs out of reality and from facing and tackling a situation, however bleak it may be."

The chapel which is large and simply designed, is open at all times for patients of any faith. Patients represent a cross section of world religions, some even being atheists. One's religion is no criterion for admission. Services are conducted regularly Sundays and on other religious holidays. Patients are free to spend time there daily if they so wish to pray or meditate. None is under compulsion to attend any time.

We mentioned earlier that beds in the ward have no curtains to be drawn around them. Why? Doctor Saunders believes that if patients can observe how peacefully other patients die, they, too, will become less fearful of their own dying. When a patient dies, family and doctor plus nurses gather around the deceased and join the prayers. The patients may participate if they so wish. The family's contact with St. Christopher's is not cut off after the patient's death. Since bereavement is so emotionally decimating, the Health Service sister follows up with home visits for as long as is necessary. On the first anniversary of the patient's death, St. Christopher's sends the family an expression of sympathy and remembrance of their loved one. As has been scientifically proven by Doctor Colin Murray Parkes in his studies of grief in adult life, the first year is usually the most traumatic.

I ended the visit with sadness at the thought of leaving, but with the hope that I would return in the near future for a longer period.

Helaine Dawson

St. Christopher's is an autonomous facility and is not connected with a medical hospital. A Canadian adaptation of the hospice concept mentioned earlier is the Palliative Care Unit at Royal Victoria Hospital, Montreal, Canada. This unit is a department of the total hospital complex. The services provided by the Palliative Care Unit are also available to other patients in the hospital as well as to home-care patients.

Ideally, the hospice is a combination of an in-patient facility and support for home care. Some groups like the New Haven, Connecticut; Montreal, Canada; and Parkwood Hospital, Canoga Park, California, hospice teams work in both areas. Some groups like Marin Hospice, Inc., Santa Barbara Hospice, and Hospice, Orange County in California, have no in-patient facilities at the present time, but they do have a staff to support home care and counsel the patient and family members. Staff anticipate problems and try to handle situations before they become emergencies. When questions arise, families can call a hospice staff member for advice. A nurse or doctor is on call and makes house visits when needed. Hospice services are provided on a twenty-four hour, seven day per week basis.

If you are interested in learning more about the hospice movement a book you can read and have on hand for referral is *The Hospice*

Movement—A Better Way To Care For The Dying by Sandol Stoddard. The author has done a great deal of research into the hospice movement and worked as a volunteer at St. Christopher's in England. The book includes information on how to start a hospice. Sandol Stoddard writes with warmth and compassion about her experiences with dying patients. In Chapter 7, she quotes Dr. Cicely Saunders:

> "You matter because you are you. You matter to the last moment of your life, and we will do all we can not only to help you die peacefully, but also to live until you die."

That statement, perhaps more than any, sums up the hospice concept. For further information about the hospice movement or for locations of hospice programs in your area, contact:

National Hospice Organization
Suite 506
301 Maple Ave. West
Vienna, Virginia 22180

Your hospital discharge planner or county social worker will also have information on support groups using a hospice approach.

At present there are no hospice facilities specifically for children. This may be due to children's need to be in familiar surroundings at home and because most parents want to keep their children at home. In some situations a hospital is the best choice, and the choice must be made on an individual basis considering all facets of the child's care and the family resources.

Home care is better for the child but more difficult for parents. Parents need a great deal of strength to go through the loss of a child and counseling may be needed for successful home care treatment. Children have little preconception of death, and go through the process easier than parents. How nice for a child to die cradled lovingly in his mother's arms, while lying on the couch watching cartoons on television, or during sleep in his own comfortable surroundings.

Home-care benefits:
1. If parents can remain calm and loving, children will have no fear of the experience.
2. Children will be less afraid of treatment at home.

3. They have the freedom to move around and play with their own toys.

4. Home care provides an opportunity for flexibility of schedule.

5. Families have time to be alone with children.

6. Being at home, families can have experiences to be treasured when the child is gone.

I traveled to the Los Angeles area to meet Dr. Jim Jett, who started a hospice project in that area. He gave me a copy of an article he wrote entitled "Taking The Hard Middle Ground," which appeared in *Medical Economics,* 1976. The following is a quote from that article.

Telling a patient or his family that there's nothing more you can do is a medical cop-out. It means you're unwilling to take the hard middle ground between aggressive treatment and pulling the curtain.

There are plenty of things you can do if you take that middle ground. Some are as old as the art of medicine itself. Others are new, the products of the developing terminal-care centers called hospices. All are geared to the premise that death, not recovery, is now the end point and that your mission is to help the patient make the most of the time he has left.

Another section of Dr. Jett's article is entitled "You Can Help Patients Give As Well As Receive." He gives an illustration of how the terminally ill can remain active. Everyone has something to give or share with others. They can express their feelings and needs with medical staff in an effort to improve care. They can help other patients, like chauffeuring someone who can no longer drive.

A chaplain friend told me that the dying patient gives him a great deal. Another friend who is a regular volunteer in a local university hospital working with the terminally ill said she learns much about living from those who are dying. She is a volunteer on call and visits patients when they need to talk, even if it is in the middle of the night. These volunteers receive specialized training before working in a hospice facility.

Our nurse, Lyn, said Larry gave her as much as she gave him. When Lyn and her husband were planning a vacation trip, Larry helped plan the route and shared some of the experiences of our trip to Bryce Canyon and Zion National Park. Larry described points of interest, best motel accommodations and restaurants, and sight-seeing routes that could be taken. Lyn had purchased a new, complicated camera for her husband as a gift for Father's Day. Larry helped select the camera and between nursing chores, he taught her how to use the camera effectively and how to take good pictures.

Larry enjoyed giving gifts to those who visited us. Sometimes it was a copy of the book he had written, or stamps he felt were a good collector's item, or a penny flattened out with the Lord's Prayer stamped on it. But mostly he gave of himself. He wrote letters and telephoned friends. Visitors told me they always felt better when they visited him. He was an inspiriting person, and it was difficult to think of him as ill.

The act of giving is therapeutic because it moves the patients' attention from concern for themselves to concern for others. And it gives families and friends the opportunity to receive, which balances out the giving-receiving cycle. Patients know they require a lot of care and their feeling of self-worth may be diminished as the need for care increases. They have much to give and we are fortunate whenever we are invited as a guest into their personal experience.

Please Remember Me

Mari Brady met Graham Banks when she went to work at Sloan-Kettering Clinic in New York. At the time, Graham did not look or act like he had cancer. He often helped her prepare for parties for the patients. Because she was young, fifteen years old, Graham felt he could talk with her. She missed his energy, warmth and humor when he was released after treatment. Graham returned again after several months and he and Mari became good friends during his hospital stay. He was again released and Mari wondered about how he was.

One day the phone rang. It was Graham's mother. She told Mari Graham was being readmitted. This time he had lost weight, was considerably weaker and they both knew he was dying. He asked Mari to write a letter, which he dictated, to his brother who had a drug problem. He and Mari had many opportunities to talk this time. Shortly before Christmas Mari accompanied him as he was carried by stretcher to a waiting ambulance. It was snowing and Graham said he looked forward to going home and to having the best Christmas ever. It was also his last, Mari wrote. His last words to her were, "Please remember me."

Mari Brady wrote a book which she entitled *Please Remember Me* in evidence of her friendship and love for Graham.

Dying patients all have a concern that they will be forgotten when they are gone. Being forgotten invalidates their existence. As long as they are remembered, they exist. The knowledge that a patient is dying provides the opportunity for families to say:

"I love you."

"Thank you for loving me."

"I'll always remember you."

or with friends:

"I've enjoyed your friendship."

"Thank you for (some event or action)"

"I'll always remember you."

No relationship is perfect but there are always things you can thank them for. If the relationship is strained for some reason, it would be better to be honest and say "Our relationship has been strained but I want you to know that I still have appreciated your friendship." Communication shows you value them as a person.

Granting Last Requests

A woman, in her seventies, had been a patient in a hospital for several weeks. Her exploratory surgery revealed widespread cancer and she was not able to go home. Each day she knew she grew weaker. She had not seen her granddaughter, who had been born a month earlier in another state. She wanted very much to see her, but she was too proud to admit to her son that she was terminally ill. She confided this to a friend, who in turn, called the son. Because the mother had not related the seriousness of her illness, he had been unaware of her need. He telephoned his mother's doctor, who confirmed the diagnosis. The son and his family were planning a motor trip during his vacation so he changed the route to include a stop to see his mother. She would never have asked him to come and even continued the pretext of temporary illness during their family visit. She tenderly held her granddaughter for long periods of time and took great interest in the return to breast-feeding. "We fed all our children that way when I was young," she explained. As they left her for the last time, she told her son, "Be sure you tell her about me."

This woman's desire to see her granddaughter was not verbalized to her son. She expressed it to her friend. It would be speculation to try to determine whether she knew her friend would arrange it. The important thing was that she got her wish—she held her granddaughter in her arms.

A terminally ill couple were re-married by a Catholic priest in a hospice unit where the husband was a patient. When they realized they were both dying of cancer, they decided this was the thing they wanted most. They had been married in a civil ceremony thirty-four years before. Both wanted the blessing of the Catholic ceremony. The wedding was held in a family room at the hospice unit. Their grown children and a dozen friends joined them in a party after the ceremony.

Last requests are unique because people are unique.

My friend, Jean Lynn, described her husband's last day to me: "It was a beautiful warm September morning. When I opened the bedroom drapes we could look out over the blue water of the bay to the hills beyond. I had picked some roses from Frank's garden and placed them in a vase next to the bed. How really blessed we were to have him close by to appreciate being home as he did in his last hours. What a lovely way to go. The morning that Frank died a Goodyear blimp went tooting along the shore line of the west bay and Frank being a naval officer and pilot in World War II, sat up and recognized it. He didn't say much but how delightful it was to share that. And then to be able to feed him a few teaspoons of yogurt so that he would go off to his new experience with a full tummy. That made me feel very gratified.

"We gave him what he needed when he needed it. He sat in the kitchen one day and decided what he wanted for his own funeral. To be able to sit in your own kitchen and look out on your own piece of land which had been developed since we had purchased it twenty years before, to be able to have everyone there when the attorney came, and being together when he died; it was very pleasant to share these things. He was in his own comfortable situation.

"We only had one rocky night before he passed on, which was, according to the old wives' tale 'the death rattle.' But was it really? You could feel the transition. I could feel his leaving. It was nothing to be afraid of. He relaxed so that he never had an emotional moment in the hour of greatest possible stress. It was just like a quiet passing, like turning the pages of a book or opening to a new chapter. It gave me such satisfaction. I never shed a tear.

"You can still rejoice in your situation because you have so much left. The spirit of having had him make the passing at home. . . the transition . . . the opening of a new experience in your own situation, an unfearful one because you feel so many qualities of the life you have shared for thirty-three years still remaining. The shell has gone on. Our shell was cremated. But the spirit of life and eternity exists in your situation because you feel that it can never leave. There was no fear in lying in the same bed. I changed the bed linens and rested on the bed where Frank had died and never felt such a sense of awe. Isn't it wonderful, I thought, that I can lie here where Frank made his transition and rejoice in the things he left for us. Many of them, material things like his garden, but the most important things were the knowledge that we had shared this great experience of life, which no one knows how or when they will have to meet. Because from life comes death and with death is a growing and a closeness and an evaluation of what you have shared. I have no feeling of his departing because so much of him is still around."

Chapter XIV

Focus on Infinity

SPIRITUALITY: THE TRANSCENDENT LIFE

"What do you do when you get to the end of the rope?" was the provocative question posed by Dr. Robert Schuller, a Los Angeles minister in a sermon that concerned itself with coping when things pile up and you cannot find an answer on a physical or an emotional level.

Dr. Oral Roberts, a well-known evangelist, put it another way in one of his sermons when he asked, "What do you do when the medicine runs out?" His question, differing slightly from Dr. Schuller's since it centers the question on the purely medical aspect, was posing the premise that there must be something more even when the medical world has no further treatment, when doctors have done all they can do.

Known as a religious healer, Dr. Roberts, who is also the founder of the Oral Roberts University, is among the growing numbers who recognize the value of treating the whole person, in body, mind and soul. Toward this concept he is building a "City of Faith" medical center complex in Tulsa, Oklahoma, which will include a sixty-story clinic, a thirty-story hospital facility and a twenty-story research center. The center will use a holistic approach, treating the body, mind and spirit of patients, and offering support to families. The emphasis of the center will be to expand the normal treatment of disease to include a strong spiritual approach.

My own experience tells me that a spiritual base is an absolute essential, not only in the role of healing, but in daily living. We feel the critical need for another source of strength when confronted with a serious illness, but crises are not necessarily limited to medical problems. Life does not exempt us from other problems just because we are ill.

The appearance of illness or injury disrupts the lives we've planned. Not all patients get physically well. Some need long-term treatment. Some die. When events happen that we cannot handle, we begin to look beyond ourselves. When our bodies do not respond to medical treatment, we must seek life on a higher level. This is not a new phenomenon. Men in all ages have found circumstances beyond their control and have sought a higher consciousness, a universal power greater than themselves. They seek the infinite when the finite world fails them.

The approach in holistic medicine is to treat the entire person—in body, mind and spirit. Scientific medicine is recognizing the truth of the existence of a spirit within man which is an integral part of the whole.

Dr. Carl Jung, one of our great psychiatrist, through years of research and study discovered certain symbols or archetypes of what he called the "collective unconscious." Dr. Jung pointed out that there is an individuation process going on in life, in which life itself seems to be striving in individuals towards wholeness, towards completeness and this individuation process is manifested or represented by a symbol which Dr. Jung calls "the mandala." It is a circular symbol, sometimes a squared circle, that appears in the myths, dreams, fairy tales and stories of races and peoples all over the world. Whenever it appears it always symbolizes a possibility of reconciliation of opposites, opposites that seemingly are irreconcilable but that come together in the life process of individuation. The individuation process indicates that a person recognizes and lives out his own unique experience of life but at the same time becomes unified with life, unified with the world, unified with mankind, and unified with God, as a culmination and fruition of this individuation process. Finite consciousness splits events into opposites: good-bad, past-future, day-night, joy-sorrow, rich-poor, health-sickness, life-death. The infinite consciousness transcends the opposites and life is lived in the freedom of higher consciousness. The opposites are only distorted views of real events. We place the "opposite" labels on them. The cycle of life includes all opposites. In our finite state we prefer one over the other—striving for life and rejecting death, for instance. In the transcendent self, we accept both life and death as a part of the perfect whole. When these opposites become integrated and harmonized, we come out with a new life. We have a sense of relationship with ourselves, with others, with life and with God.

One of the pairs of opposites that gives us a great deal of trouble is the past-future one. We either want to live in the past and relive old experiences or we long for something in the future. We regret things that happened in the past and worry about what may happen in the future. We want to be well as we were in the past, or young like we were, or we spend our time and energy wishing we were married or unmarried, through school or on a vacation or a myriad of other desired goals or events. When energy is spent on worry or desire for the past or the future, we miss the only real life we have, that in the NOW. The opposites create tension and anxiety. This is a providential state, which forces us from our reliance on ourselves to a search for a higher power. The now is a transcendent state, free of the tensions of the opposites, a state in which we find the only true peace and joy.

Another pair of opposites that can cause conflict are the active-passive roles we assume. On one hand we actively try to manage our lives alone and on the other, we passively sit back and wait for someone else to solve our problems, i.e. the doctor, minister, or on a higher level, God. We try to resist illness, to either deny it exists or become intent on fighting it. Or we try to cope—a kind of putting up with the situation with little expectation that it will change. We can acquiesce—with a "well, that's the way it is" attitude. We can accept it all, either as a positive attitude of the realization of the situation or negatively as a kind of giving up.

We can try to run our own lives. If we are successful, we can take all the credit. But what happens when our lives become a total disaster, become unmanageable, and we can no longer handle situations and problems? What happens when we try to run our own lives and fail?

This is an awakening, a realization that leads us to seek help and look for a higher power, greater than ourselves. When we become free of the opposites, we can be active and passive as the situation requires, but not locked into either extreme. We can do all we can on a finite level but attuned to the Divine Order of the universal infinite.

Dr. Richard Carlson is the medical director of an alcoholic rehabilitation center in Redwood City, California. I discussed with him the problem of alcoholism as it relates to terminal illness. In my research for this book I found many cases in which the patients or family members used alcohol to escape the reality and hopelessness of illness.

"Alcoholism itself is a terminal illness," he said. "As a matter of fact, alcoholism is a process of dying—you are not living."

All through this book I have placed an emphasis on attitude, how you view your situation. Even when a circumstance cannot be changed, when our attitude changes, our lives also change. Dr. Carlson said that behind every attitude is a thought or consideration. We deny a reality. We decide: "This just isn't so," "I don't have cancer," "I'm not an alcoholic," "I'm not getting old," when the reality proves just the opposite. Dr. Carlson calls this: "This isn't it."

"Our misery comes out of that, because as long as this is not it," he said, "we can do nothing but resist. That is all we are given to do. As soon as you accept 'this is it,' then you begin manifesting that acceptance. And out of acceptance comes happiness and satisfaction. Acceptance has a quality of expansion to it.

"The attitude has to do with all of it. It is as though there were a lightness about it, with people who really do trust—who have their faith and trust in a higher power. They are light about it, they are willing, they accept it. And having accepted, they lighten up. When they are resisting, and when they are worrying about it, when they are coming from this isn't it, they are definitely upset. And they are tight. They're unhappy. They are suffering. A letting go of, or an acceptance of, any chronic illness can change the condition in which that chronic illness is held, from one of suffering and misery to one of acceptance and lightness and happiness. It doesn't matter what it is. Sickness or health, or suffering, even death itself."

The same principle was at work at the Center for Attitudinal Healing in Tiburon using the process of children helping other children. I asked Dr. Carlson if he felt this was an effective approach to dealing with illness. He replied: "Absolutely. You cannot do it alone. And the amazing thing is whatever you discover on your own, if you share that, then it becomes real. And of course somebody else takes it up and it becomes a new and different experience, which becomes real to them and they share it— in this way the whole process grows. But the becoming enlightened at any level is a "so what" unless it manifests itself in your life, unless you carry it out in the world and really share it.''

Many situations develop in life that appear "bad," "hopeless," or "miserable." They can also be described as "hitting bottom." From one perspective they are to be avoided; from another they can be a blessing.

Spiritual pilgrimages begin in a variety of ways—most often unsought, as an interruption in a neatly planned, comfortable life— and often out of crisis.

Ernest Gordon had another kind of "bad" experience. He wanted to escape from a Japanese prison camp. He would not have chosen captivity. And the Japanese soldiers were not aware that they would play a role in bringing about circumstances in which God could change the direction of Ernest Gordon's life. He describes his experiences in a book called *Through the Valley of the Kwai.*

The story begins when Ernest Gordon wakened from a pleasant dream of past events to the reality of the Death House, as it was called, when two orderlies dumped a tenth body on the floor next to him. The Death House was supposed to be a hospital, but men came there to die, to escape the horrors of life in the camp. As the orderlies left, taking the lamp with them, Ernest Gordon settled back in darkness and wondered why he had to end up in such a place.

He thought of his pleasant university life in Scotland, the happiness of sailing, and the first appearance of rumors of war. Although a disability due to an injury kept him out of the military for awhile, he eventually joined up, enlisting in the 93rd Highlands because he didn't want a desk job. In 1942, his regiment crossed a causeway connecting the Malayan Peninsula with Singapore, and proceeded down the straits to Sumatra and a coastal city of Padang. It became apparent that Padang would be taken by the Japanese so the British officers devised a plan whereby some of them would try to escape by getting to a fishing village north of Padang. They also needed someone to sail them to Ceylon, about 1200 miles away. The voyage began hopefully but ended with the appearance of a heavily armed Japanese tanker. Their capture resulted in three and a half years of imprisonment.

As life deteriorated in the series of camps, the men learned to survive by the law of the jungle; only the strongest would survive. You looked out for yourself—made the best deal you could—got the best camp job (servers of food could short the others to get a larger portion themselves, for instance), no mercy was shown the dying, the ill were ignored for fear of getting the disease and hate prevailed: hate for the Japanese, themselves, other camp

members and God. Some men had turned to religion when they were captured but dropped it when it had not supported them and the situation
worsened. Once in awhile two men might form a friendship, but then one of
them would disappear. They learned to avoid forming friendships.

Ernest Gordon became ill with diphtheria and entered the Death House.
He called this "the lowest level of life." Conditions were so bad in the hospital (bed bugs, stench, uncleanliness and the sound of dying), that he asked
to be moved to the morgue because it was quiet and relatively cleaner. He
slept on the dirt floor. The guards let him move into the morgue because
they expected him to be a corpse soon anyway.

The turning point in his illness and in his life came when a friend arranged
to build a little isolation hut so he could be moved from the Death House.
Doctors concurred that there was nothing more medically they could do,
and concluded that the isolation hut would work as a safeguard to protect
others in the camp from his disease. They also agreed that he could have a
decent end there—they also expected him to die.

Mr. Gordon rejected the idea of dying but being realistic, decided he
would like to write his parents. This is what he wrote:

Dear Mum and Dad,

If one of my friends passes this on to you it will mean that I've guessed
wrongly and that I'm not coming back. I'm sorry. I'd have made it if I
could. When I escaped, first from Singapore and then from Sumatra, I
thought I was bound to return to you safely.

Don't have any regrets. I suppose it just couldn't have been otherwise.
I've enjoyed life. I'm glad I was brought up in the country with the sea at
the front of the house and the hills at the back. I'm glad I had you as
parents. If I seldom showed any sign of appreciation for all the love and
kindness you've given me, it was because I took it too much for granted that
this is the way life is. I know it isn't always that way, now. Accept a "Thank
You" from me to you, please!

I've enjoyed all the things I've ever done. Even those things I should have
done better.

That summer before the war was absolutely wizard. I should have spent
more time with you and less time sailing. But you'll forgive me for that, I
know, because you liked sailing, too.

I think there's over a hundred pounds in the bank at Innellan, another
forty or so in the Hong Kong and Shanghai Bank of Singapore, and maybe
the Army will chip in what pay I have coming to me.

Take it and have a good vacation in the South of England. Stay at a hotel
where your breakfast will be served in bed. You'll make me happy if you do
this.

There's a great deal of good about life that will never die. There's a goodness at the heart of it, I believe.

Pass on my love to my friends, and be assured of mine for you, always. Kiss Grace and Pete for me.

Bless you!

Aye yours,
Ernest

He gave the letter to a friend in case he didn't make it. Then he thought, "Going to die, was I? I found myself resisting the whole idea. I recalled the faces and solemn words of Eliza Doolittle, 'Not bloodly likely!' when, for me, was not now. The battle between life and death goes on all the time," I said to myself. "Life has to be cherished, not let go. I have made up my mind. I am not going to surrender."

Then I asked myself, "What do I do about it?" It was a voice other than reason that replied, 'You could live. You could be. There's a purpose you have to fulfill. You'll become more conscious of it every day that you keep on living. There's a task for you; a responsibility that is yours and only yours.' "Good enough," I said to myself, "I'll get on with it."

The clean hut lifted his spirits. A friend came and gave him his first bath since he became ill. The friend also brought food and cared for his legs, which had become infected. Another camp member began to share Gordon's care. Strength began to return to the body and finally some sensation returned to his paralyzed legs. He began his own program of physical therapy.

The atmosphere in the camp began to change as men began to care about each other. Ernest Gordon began to realize that there was another form of healing—healing that came from God. He began to study the New Testament, and he and a few other men got together to discuss their knowledge of God in relation to their experience. They discovered the power of love and the joy of giving. They discovered the strength of unity and the complete satisfaction in fulfilling a Divine Purpose. "Not to be served, but to serve."

They formed groups to visit the sick. They fashioned an artificial leg from scraps of material and metal from cans. They started having classes in history, philosophy, economics, math, sciences and languages. They shared the few books they had. They formed an orchestra using some instruments the men had kept with them when they were captured, and some they fashioned from bamboo. Their Japanese captors attended performances given by the orchestra, sitting in front row seats. The men also got together for community singing and dramatic performances. They extended their inner spiritual change to an outer social change. They found life—and freedom during their captivity. They no longer viewed the Japanese as "the enemy" and cared for Japanese wounded as they did their own.

Ernest Gordon took what he learned in the camp, about life and death and the power of love and the Divine Purpose back into the world when the war ended and he was released.

He completed graduate studies at the Hartford Theological Seminary. He was so deeply touched by the young men who died in the prison camp that he wanted to work with young people. Less than a year after he accepted his first ministerial post, his dream of working with youth became a reality, and he became Dean of the Chapel at Princeton University. Even his writing of the book, *Through the Valley of the Kwai,* published by Harper and Row in 1962, was an effort to share his discoveries.

The following is a quote from the end of that book:

"Here I found that although prison camp and campus were poles apart, many of the questions asked me were identical to those I had been called upon to answer in Southeast Asia. The miracle I knew in the jungle was being repeated daily on the campus—the miracle of God at work in His world.

I recalled that when I was at Paisley I had been told how the old-time weavers, all the while they were making their beautiful and intricate patterns, saw no more than the backs of their shawls. Nothing was visible to them but a tangle of colored threads. They never saw the design they were creating until they took the finished fabric from their looms.

The parallel to the mortal lot is plain. Human experience appears to us—as the shawls did to the weavers—to be no more than incomprehensible tangles of colored threads, whereas in fact life represents the ordered threads in a great design—the design being woven daily on the loom of eternity. Looking back, in all the chaos and confusion, I could see a splendid purpose being worked out.

In my time of decision, nature and reason were neutral. They did not speak to me of anything that made possible a significant understanding of myself and my fellow man. They did not show me the vision of the Infinitely Great.

Jesus, however, had spoken to me, had convinced me of the love of God, and had drawn me into a meaningful fellowship with other men as brothers. Because of him I had come to see the world in a new way as the creation of God—not purposeless but purposeful.

He had opened me to life and life to me.

In the prison camp we had discovered nothing new. The grace we had experienced is the same in every generation and must ever be received afresh.

The good news for man is that God, in Christ, has shared his suffering; for that is what God is like. He has not shunned the responsibility of freedom. He shares in the saddest and most painful experiences of His children, even that experience which seems to defeat us all, death itself.

He comes into our Death House to lead us through it."

The question "Why?" is repeated over and over in books and in my encounters with people in crisis. Sometimes it takes the form of

"Why now?" "Why here?" or "Why me?" But the why is always there.

In *The Matthew Tree* by H. T. Wright (a pseudonym), the author describes how she and her mother sat and waited at her father's bedside after he suffered a stroke. He had been in a coma and they wanted to be with him when he regained consciousness. His first words were "Why?—"Why?" The author writes a truthful, humorous, agonizing, human and touching book about the seven-year duration of his illness.

Joni Eareckson in her book *Joni* describes how she questioned "Why?" when she was paralyzed from the neck down in a swimming accident just at the time she was planning to attend college.

The question "Why?" is always a spiritual one. "Why me, Lord?" It usually is followed by "What have I done to deserve this?" In back of this question is our assumption that we are in total control of our lives. We would not plan illness, injury, scandal, failure, poverty, or any kind of adversity. That's not the "good life" we're promised in advertising, in movies and books. As children, we learned "and they lived happily ever after!" And we believed that meant adversity-free lives. But life is not one-sided—it is made up of opposites. For everything there is a season or a time. And we do not set the time or place—God does. And we don't have control over our lives.

Everything that happens in this world happens at the time God chooses.
He sets the time for birth and
    the time for death,
the time for planting and the
    time for pulling up,
the time for killing and the
    time for healing,
the time for tearing down and
    the time for building.
He sets the time for sorrow
    and the time for joy,
the time for mourning and the
    time for dancing,
the time for making love and
    the time for not making love,

the time for kissing and the
    time for not kissing.
He sets the time for finding
    and the time for losing,
the time for saving and the
    time for throwing away,
the time for tearing and the
    time for mending,
the time for silence and the
    time for talk.
He sets the time for love and
    the time for hate,
the time for war tnd the time
    for peace.

Ecclesiastes 3 (Today's English Version)

And God does not bring adversity into our lives as punishment. On a mortal level we may view it as punishment—as being unjust—but God brings all the experiences of our lives to us to make us grow closer to Him. If we could successfully run our own lives we wouldn't need God.

Chaplains and Ministers

If you already have a religious belief and your life is grounded in the faith that religion brings, then that religious faith acts as a channel through which all of life flows. Larry and I shared in a belief that all events of life are meant to help us grow and learn, that they were a challenge, an experience of learning. Therefore, his illnesses and my nursing care were just experiences in a *process* of growing—a process which we totally trusted.

At night, when I crawled into bed beside him, I was comforted by his closeness. In the darkness of the night, I reached over and put my hand in his. He was there. Sometimes my only prayer before dropping off into an exhausted sleep was, "Thank you, God, that we can be together." But at other times Larry would end the day with a prayer. This one is typical.

Our Dear Father:

We thank you for the gift of another day—

A day during which we've had opportunities for being together and having encounters with other people. A chance to feel within and to express without, our love for our children and our grandson—for each other and for YOU. We are more than ever grateful to You for the gift of life and for this holy time in which we can know and experience love. We pray that You will make more and more of this love available to us, through Your Grace, and that we will come to experience more wonder and appreciation for life and love as we experience it here on earth. We recognize we are finite and limited people lapsing into egocentric, self-centered behavior at any and all times. We ask for Your help in transcending these limitations and entering more fully into the Kingdom of the We—Your Eternal Life, where we are never alone but joined to You.

We pray for Your forgiveness for our shortcomings and ask for Your love which heals us and makes us whole. Teach us how to serve You where we are.

Amen.

Since Larry was an American Baptist Minister, we had many friends in the ministry. Sometimes Larry would call them; sometimes they would call him. Former Chaplain Byron Eshelman, now retired from the prison chaplaincy, first met Larry when Larry was a prisoner in San Quentin. Their friendship continued when Larry was in seminary and during his ministry. He followed the many turns and twists of Larry's illness, visiting him both in the hospital and at home. Many of their conversations were theologically- oriented. They often discussed the ideas of Fritz Kunkel which were taught in the School of Religion at San Quentin, when Byron was Chaplain and Larry was a prisoner. Kunkel's teachings were based on the idea that it is only through crisis that you grow and mature, that God brings crisis into our lives to make us grow. We would never choose a crucifixion or the bleak, dismal happenings of life: the prison, the cancer, the scandal, the so- called unhappy experiences of life. But it is only through crisis and the crucifixion that the resurrection can come.

Larry found meaning and growth in his prison experiences at San Quentin. His first book, *Return To The World,* was an expression of this. His second unpublished manuscript describes his feeling that cancer was a blessing. This belief, this faith in the meaning of adversity, sustained us.

Dr. Cecil Osborne, former pastor of the First Baptist Church in Burlingame and now working with Yokefellows, Inc., called, wrote and visited Larry through the years. It was Dr. Osborne who sponsored Larry when he was released from prison.

Rev. Robert Paulus, another minister friend, faithfully visited Larry. Bob could relate to Larry's illnesses and surgeries because he was seriously injured when he was pinned between his own vehicle and a van that hit him. Bob came very close to dying and although he recuperated, he had many surgeries to repair damage done by that accident. He and Larry shared their feelings of finiteness and suffering.

Rev. Charles Walker graduated from the same seminary as Larry and was supportive of Larry's prison ministry for many years. He came to visit and often brought his guitar and sang and played religious songs, which he wrote.

Psychological and religious counseling was continuous, but never in a programmed, scheduled way. It happened naturally, and Larry was often doing the "counseling."

Ministers and chaplains are available in a hospital setting to help people in a medical crisis. I visited with Chaplain Warren Dale at Mills Memorial Hospital in San Mateo. I asked him to explain the role of the chaplain. He said, "The chaplain's role differs according to training, skill, interest, and job description. Most chaplains provide pastoral support which includes visits, sacraments, and prayer. Some are available to visit the patient at home. They often provide spiritual counseling involving questions of meaning, clarification, alienation, forgiveness, and bereavement.

It is beyond spiritual counseling that chaplains will differ. Some are trained to help families respond to the emotional stages of illness, of death and of dying. Some are trained in social work, pastoral or family counseling, and offer brief counseling in those fields.

Chaplains also differ in their relationship with the hospital and thus their familiarity and influence with the health-care team. Some chaplains are full- or part-time employees of the hospital and thus have an opportunity to develop a relationship with the hospital administration, medical, and hospital staff (physicians, nurses, and other care givers). Some chaplains are supported by foundations, parishes, task forces, or churches. They too can develop a relationship with some medical and hospital staff.

Other chaplains cover the hospital by a rotational system and may be more denominationally oriented. These chaplains may also have a relationship with some staff but their role is usually limited to pastoral support.

In addition to the chaplaincy service another important group available in many hospitals is the volunteer emotional support group. Some are called auxiliary support service, parachaplains, department of pastoral care, or chaplain assistants. These volunteers assist the chaplain in supporting patients and their families.

There is, however, one more common and most valuable resource offered by most chaplains; they can listen, help clarify, and often refer the patient or family to the needed resource in the hospital or community.

Chaplains do not visit every patient, respecting the privacy of patients and realizing that not every patient wants a visit. Some patients have ministers, priests or rabbis from their own faith who visit. Some patients have no interest in religious matters and feel they can handle their illness on their own. Chaplains therefore usually see patients or families when a visit is requested. A patient may make the request, medical staff may refer the patient to the chaplain or families and friends may telephone for assistance.

Some chaplains work closely with medical staff and are considered part of the "crisis team" and may be called upon to assist with patients and families in an emergency room, intensive care unit, or surgical area, places where trauma is most likely to exist.

Chaplains often speak to community groups, assist in community programs involving illness and dying, and provide in-service training for doctors, nurses and other medical staff.

I feel chaplains offer a great service to patients and families. I am very grateful Larry and I had the support of so many chaplains and ministers. It can be lonely in a hospital waiting room if you try to handle everything yourself. The warmth and comfort of a chaplain or volunteer can make the experience bearable. Sometimes a patient or family member needs an objective other person to talk with, someone who understands the emotional upheaval going on in their lives.

As Warren Dale said, "Emotional support from a trained listener is an element that can help turn a most difficult crisis into a special experience of growth. It need only be sought and requested by the person in need."

I went to Peninsula Hospital in Burlingame, California to visit with an old friend, Chaplain Walter Johnson. I stepped off the elevator onto the third floor and approached the door marked Chaplain. The door was slightly ajar and I could hear Walt ending a conversation on the telephone. Walt knew Larry through their ministries and we sometimes meet each other at conferences, since our interests are parallel. Walt smiled and greeted me. "I hoped you would be late," he said. "I need about ten minutes of quiet before we talk." "That's fine with me," I replied. "I could use the time to relax, too." He went into another office and I stayed in the large main room.

The soft background music was a pleasant contrast to the still, empty, and quiet third floor hospital atmosphere. I sat near the window and closed my eyes, feeling the warmth of the sun releasing the tension of the day. Walt had said he wanted only ten minutes quiet time, but had been in his office only a couple of minutes when the phone rang for the first of three incoming calls during that ten-minute period. He asked me to answer the phone and take messages. The third call I took sounded important and when he returned to the main office I gave him the message. He picked up the phone and spoke to someone within the hospital. He ended with, "I'll be right down, I want to meet him."

He asked me to accompany him and, wanting to be sure this was a real invitation and not just a polite gesture, I offered to wait in the office. "Come along," he said. "I think you'll enjoy seeing this man." On the way down in the elevator, Walt explained that the man we would be seeing traveled a long distance for treatment. He stayed temporarily at a nearby motel, but Walt hoped to find him a room in a home. The man had cancer, both his legs had been amputated just above the knee and he wore prostheses.

The older man smiled at us as we entered the room. He was sitting comfortably in a waiting room area between medical offices and treatment rooms. The nurses moved chairs so that we could join him. Walt discussed the man's living accommodations and said he had been making contacts with individuals in the community and was waiting for some return calls. The man was most appreciative but seemed more intent on telling us about his adventurous day than he was interested in discussing his housing. He had driven a long way from his home to the hospital that day and had been late (he said apologetically) because he had trouble with the fuel pump on his car. He quickly added that people stopped to assist him, that he had the car repaired and was only two hours late for his appointment for treatment. A doctor walked in during his telling the story about his car, and the doctor quipped, "You're in better shape than your car!" We all laughed and I was grateful for a doctor who could share in the conversation and who had a sense of humor. The man hoisted himself up on his artificial legs by using two canes. The last sight I had of him was as he went out the door and along the surrounding sidewalk, loping off distance with great long strides.

Walt and I went back upstairs to his office and talked for over an hour about his work, but nothing he said could compare with the experience of seeing him at work.

Walt explained how he viewed his role as chaplain, "I found out that the most creative things happen when I try my best to be human, meet people in their humanness, and affirm that humanness, through just tuning in—that I call loving people. To me, love is really allowing my life to attune with your life, and to really pay attention to you, and what your concern is, your thoughts, your feelings, and struggles. I become a guest in your planet, your world of experience and feeling. Then as a guest in your experience, to be a resource person in any way you want to use me."

We talked about some of the difficult decisions that patients need to make while in the hospital. "They have a choice," he said. "They not only have a choice, but they have lots of options and lots of help. If the medical staff knows that they have those wants, they will try to fill them. If they feel you want advice, they give advice. So it really starts with the patient and the family expressing what they really want.

"It's good to ask the doctor, 'What should I do,' to get his opinion, if it helps you get more information in order to make your decision. But I don't think people are very happy leading their lives according to somebody else's plan. Now you may have to do all kinds of things you don't want to do, because that's the way the cards are dealt. Your options may be somewhat limited. But even within that framework, it's still your life and you have to live it the best way you can. A support team helps the family do it the way it's best for the family. The family really maintains the control and the responsibility, not the consultants or the resource people."

One of the things a chaplain does is comfort people. I asked Walt how he does this. He explained, "I'll give you my definition of comfort. Comfort is quite different from what most people think it is. Most people think that comfort is saying, 'There, there, it's going to be all right, Evelyn. You just see this through. I know it's miserable now, but it's going to be all right.' Comfort (from Latin) has been twisted. We usually think of the person being weak, that we will bring our strength to the person.

The Latin prefix C O M means '*with.*' And the F O R T is from *forte,* meaning 'strength.' Comfort literally means 'with strength.' So when I comfort a person, I depend on, count on, and know that deep within them, are strengths that they are not aware of, that they will discover as we talk about what is really going on. I can confront them with a reality. We can face the realities together. And I know that if we face the realities together in an atmosphere of love and caring, that strength is going to come from within them."

Dr. Ernle Young, Chaplain at the Stanford Medical Center, also spent some time with me discussing the role of a chaplain. I have heard Ernle speak to community groups on topics such as medical ethics, euthanasia, and bereavement. When Larry was unable to perform a wedding ceremony for our son, Ernle officiated at the ceremony.

Ernle expressed many of the same views of the chaplaincy as the other chaplains. Ernle explained that the medical center gets many patients who come from out of town. He tries to give them priority in visiting because they have no community support. Older people typically have fewer friends. Families with very young children often need support, as do those who have terminal diagnoses. When patients get close to death, the spiritual questions loom larger and larger, "especially questions about forgiveness and what happens after death," he explained.

I asked Ernle what he learns from the patients. "I learn so many things. I learn to order my own life, my own priorities. Seeing a terminal patient reminds me that I could die tonight; that if I were in his or her position, I would want everything to be as it should be, and this I want for myself. And secondly, how important it is to live fully and meaningfully, with all my relationships straight and clear. I learn a lot about faith—faith as in trusting (not faith so much as believing in miracles)—in trusting, really letting go and saying, 'This is the mess that I'm in and I put it in your hands, God.' And I learn an enormous amount about courage. What the human spirit is capable of. About living as best you possibly can to maximize each day. To make each day count."

Many people begin praying when they are in crisis and they want God to step in and handle a situation they cannot handle themselves. They not only request help but they outline specifically how they want the situation resolved. Effective prayer must acknowledge God's supremacy, and have an expression of gratitude. Prayer must be free of limitations on God as to how He will answer.

When Larry worked at San Quentin he brought home a prayer which had been mimeographed and left in the chapel. The author is unknown.

ANSWERED PRAYER

I asked God for strength, that I might achieve;
    I was made weak, that I might learn humbly to obey . . .
I asked for health, that I might do greater things;
    I was given infirmity, that I might do better things . . .

I asked for riches, that I might be happy;
  I was given poverty that I might be wise . . .
I asked for power, that I might have the praise of men;
  I was given weakness, that I might feel the need of God. . .
I asked for all things, that I might enjoy life;
  I was given life, that I might enjoy all things . . .
I got nothing that I asked for—but everything I had hoped for.
  Almost despite myself, my unspoken prayers were answered.
I am, among all men, most richly blessed.

Another article, author or source unknown, also came from San Quentin. It meant much to me during Larry's illness. It helped me remember the meaning of our experience.

THE DISAPPOINTMENTS OF LIFE

"THIS THING IS FROM ME"
(I Kings 12:24)

The disappointments of life are in reality only the decrees of love. I have a message for thee today, my child. I will whisper it softly in thine ear, in order that the storm clouds which appear may be gilt with glory, and that the thorns on which thou mayest have to walk be blunted. The message is but short—a tiny sentence—but allow it to sink into the depths of thine heart, and be to thee as a cushion on which to rest thy weary head: "This thing is from Me."

Hast thou never thought that all which concerns thee, concerns Me also? He that toucheth thee toucheth the apple of Mine eyes (Zech. 2:28). Thou hast been precious in Mine eyes, that is why I take a special interest in thine upbringing. When temptation assails thee, and the "enemy comes in like a flood"—I would wish thee to know that "This thing is from Me." I am the God of circumstances. Thou hast not been placed where thou art by chance, but it is because it is the place I have chosen for you. Didst thou not ask to become humble? Behold, I have placed thee in the very place where this lesson is to be learned. It is by thy surroundings and thy companions that the working of My will is to come about.

Hast thou money difficulties? Is it hard to keep within thine income? "This thing is from Me." For I am He that possesseth all things. I wish thee to draw everything from Me, and that thou depend entirely on Me. My riches are illimitable (Phil. 4:19). Put my promise to the proof, so that it may not be said of thee, "Yet in this thing ye did not believe the Lord thy God."

Art thou passing through a night of affliction? "This thing is from Me." I am the Man of sorrows and acquainted with grief (Isa. 53:3). I have left thee without human support that in turning to Me thou mightest obtain eternal consolation (2 Thess. 2:16-17).

Has some friend disappointed thee? One to whom thou hadst opened thine heart? "This thing is from Me." I have allowed this disappointment that thou mightest learn that the best Friend is Jesus. He preserves us from falling, fights for us in our combats; yea, the best friend is Jesus. I long to be thy confidant.

Has someone said false things of thee? Leave that, and come to Me, under My wings, away from the place of wordy dispute, "for I will bring forth thy righteousness as the Light, and thy judgment as the noonday" (Ps. 37:6). Have thy plans been all upset? Art thou crushed and weary? "This thing is from Me." Hast thou made plans and then coming, asked me to bless them? I wish to make thy plans for thee. I will take the responsibility, for it is too heavy for thee, thou couldst not perform it alone (Ex. 18:18). Thou are *but an instrument* and *not an agent*.

Hast thou desired fervently to do some great work for Me? Instead of that thou hast laid on one side, on a bed of sickness and suffering. "This thing is from Me." I was unable to attract thine attention whilst thou wast so active. I wish to teach thee some of My deep lessons. It is only those who have learned to wait patiently who can serve Me. My greatest workers are sometimes those who are laid from active service in order that they may learn to wield the weapon of prayer.

Art thou suddenly called to occupy a difficult position full of responsibilities? Go forward, counting on Me. I am giving thee the position full of responsibilities and difficulties for the reason that Jehovah thy God will bless thee in all thy works, and in all the business of thy hands (Deut. 15:18). This day I place in thy hand a pot of holy oil. Draw from it freely, My child, that all the circumstances arising along the pathway, each word that gives thee pain, each interruption trying to thy patience, each manifestation of thy feebleness, may be anointed with this oil. *Remember* that interruptions are divine instructions. The sting will go in the measure in which thou seest *Me* in all things. Therefore, set your heart unto all the works that I testify among you this day. For it is your life (Deut. 32:46-47).

Spirituality, a belief in the supremacy of God, had been a focal point of our lives long before Larry became ill. We felt that we were led to be together, that Larry was divinely led to become a minister and to pursue a career in his ministry. It was only natural that we also believed that his illness was a learning experience and that we were meant to discover new meaning from that experience as well as all the others.

Awareness, creativity, spontaneity, intimacy in relationships, and joy are by-products of an abandonment, a spiritual transcendence into a state of consciousness free of egocentric tension. We are not aware of the reality of life if we are caught up in worry or fear. We cannot be truly creative or spontaneous if our thoughts are oriented into old patterns of living and methods of problem solving. We cannot have intimacy in relationships with others until we are free of our own self-centered needs and goals. Joy is an emotion that only comes from our real Self.

Giving is a spiritual quality. We can only give if we are aware of another's need, and have the resources to respond. Giving comes from concern about another person, and concern is a form of love. Love is the most positive emotion, and is the greatest spiritual quality. It has the potential to change lives and to change the world. Giving is an expression of love. Everyone has something to give and to share; and the greatest, most long-lasting gift we can give to another is a spiritual one.

Patients, families, friends, medical staff and community groups have unique knowledge, experiences, talent, and concern to share with each other. Together they make up a team, a "we," and are stronger as a group than as individuals.

I use a daily devotional guide. For me it works best if I read it early in the morning. The devotions are short and take little time to read but they set the tone for the day for me. Many times the daily messages seem inspired to answer problems or questions in my life. Sometimes they provide insight needed to help me grow spiritually. I use Unity's "Daily Word" simply because I like the format best. The Upper Room, Secret Place, and Alcoholics Anonymous "Twenty Four Hours a Day" are a few other daily devotional guides available in churches, religious bookstores and through Alcoholics Anonymous.

We used meditations for Larry for relaxation and pain control. I found that I could do meditations myself while doing dishes, cooking, doing laundry and while sitting in a hot tub of water and bathing, eliciting both physical and mental relaxation. Meditation made two important contributions in my life; *emptying out* the anxiety, stress, physical tiredness and worry thought patterns that accumulated during the day and from the silence of meditation came *the filling up* with energy, strength (physical and emotional) and a clarity of mind.

Prayer also has an *emptying* and *filling up* process on the spiritual level. Prayer is a communication of thoughts and feelings to God and a quiet listening for His communication back to me. There is a lot of similarity between the process of meditation and prayer and sometimes I found they overlapped. Meditation is a form of altered consciousness, extended thought patterns or reflections. I always began with a meditation because I was caught up in the busy affairs of the world all day and until I emptied out that thought pattern, I was not fit for a spiritual level prayer petition to God. There is a sense, however, in which every thought is a prayer because God hears everything—meditation used preparatory to prayer clears the channel and improves intensity in the prayer process.

We live on two levels, simultaneously, in our physical and emotional form and in our spirit. The spiritual God-center provides the real life for all parts. By retreating into meditation and prayer I could empty out all the frustration of the "pressure-cooker" world, fill up with the tranquility of the other world (the only reality), enabling me to re-enter the "pressure-cooker" world with needed power and clarity. They are not either-or worlds where I swing like a pendulum from one to the other but rather a continuous flow so the two are merged into one abundant life. There are many books on prayer and meditation. Three I use are:

Escape to Reality by Thomas H. Troeger
The Art of Meditation by Joel S. Goldsmith
Clarity In Prayer by David C. Jacobsen

Unity's "Daily Word" is available by writing:
  Daily Word
  Unity Village, Missouri 64065
Unity also has a twenty-four hour per day telephone service for their Silent Unity prayer center if you need to talk with someone. The number is (816) 524-5104. If you have an urgent spiritual need and have no means of paying for the call, you may call toll free 800-821-2935 (this does not include Alaska, Hawaii or Missouri). Many other churches and religious groups have a twenty-four hour telephone counseling service. (Suicide Prevention Bureau and crisis lines of all kinds are available. Suicide Prevention will be listed in your telephone directory. Check with your local church or Council

of Churches office for other crisis line information.) Add these numbers to your emergency phone list.

The following is an excerpt from a tape Larry made, "Meditation On The Opposites."

"Life is constantly bringing us into crisis. Byron Eshelman, who was Chaplain at San Quentin, gave a sermon called the Vinedresser, in which he makes a point that through all the experiences of life God is constantly pruning us. Through all the experiences of life this pruning process goes on and of course it's like when you prune a rose bush, you cut it right back to nothing in order for it to develop beautiful blossoms. So life is doing that to us, through the individuation process, through the pruning process that Byron Eshelman mentions in his sermon. Life is constantly drawing us into "doghouse" experiences, the ones we would like to avoid. Ultimately, unto death itself, which is the great crisis of life. Of course the extreme opposites of life are life and death. Death is with us from the time we are born. We develop new ways of looking at life and death that enable us to transcend, to reconcile, to harmonize these opposites and come out into a new kind of life. It's the resurrected life. It's the life beyond the cross, a life that is free of finite opposites. When you reach this state I am talking about, it is a state of abandonment. It's a condition of trusting God, Providence, the Vinedresser, the Pruner.

As far as your life is concerned, your life is not your own. We have this business of believing that our life belongs to us. Our life does not belong to us. We say, 'Well it's my life and I can do what I want to do with it.' But the Bible and the theological perspective on life and especially my own experience, leads me to understand that despite every appearance to the contrary, I do not run my own life: God is in complete control.

The ego is not God. When you find your Self, you find God. When you realize that God controls your life, you have confidence, you have faith that God knows what you need, that God has a plan for your life. God has ordained and predestined everything that has happened to you—including illness.

Ultimately He chooses for you things that you would never choose; to help you grow spiritually, to help you mature, to help you enter into the Kingdom, to focus on infinity, to help you realize that God is in you,

you are in God,

and all is well."

Bibliography

Acterberg, J., O.C. and Stephanie Matthews Simonton. *Stress, Psychological Factors and Cancer.* New Medicine Press, 1976.

Airola, Paavo. *How To Get Well.* Health Plus, Publishers, 1974.

American Cancer Society. "Service and Rehabilitation—Home Health Care Programs."

"Ardent Booster of Holistic Health." *San Francisco Chronicle,* September 12, 1978.

Baer, Louis Shattuck. *Let The Patient Decide.* Philadelphia: Westminster Press, 1978.

Banashek, Susan. "Family, The Best Medicine." *San Francisco Chronicle,* May 11, 1976.

Baulch, Lawrence (Rev.). *All Streams Run To The Sea.* Evelyn M. Baulch, 1977.

Bell, John. "Miracle Cancer Cures That Show There's Always Hope." *National Enquirer,* February 27, 1979.

Benowicz, Robert J. *Non-Prescription Drugs and Their Side Effects.* New York: Grosset and Dunlap, 1977.

Benson, Herbert. *The Relaxation Response.* New York: William Morrow, 1975.

Berne, Eric. *Games People Play.* New York: Grove Press, 1964.

Brady Mari. *Please Remember Me.* New York: Doubleday, 1977.

"Body's Own Painkillers." *San Mateo Times,* August 28, 1978.

Breecher, Maury. "Simple No Drug Technique Can Help 67 Million Sufferers." *National Enquirer,* November 14, 1978.

Bricklin, Mary. *Natural Healing.* Emmaus, PA: Rodale Press, Inc., 1976.

Brody, Jane E. with Arthur I. Holleb. *You Can Fight Cancer and Win.* New York: Quadrangle/The New York Times Book Co., 1977.

Brown, Barbara B. *New Mind, New Body. Biofeedback: New Directions for the Mind.* New York: Harper and Row, 1974.

Brown, Cathy. "New No Medication Technique Relieves Pain of Arthritis." *National Enquirer,* August 29, 1978.

Buber, Martin. *I and Thou.* New York: Scribner, 1970.

Bunyan, John. *The Pilgrim's Progress,* Porter and Coates.

Cardiopulmonary Resuscitation, The American National Red Cross, 1967.

Carroll, Jerry. "Thoughts with Death at Hand." *San Francisco Chronicle,* August 20, 1978.

Carter, Michelle. "Letting the World Know How You Want to Die." *San Mateo Times,* November 8, 1978.

Carter, Michelle. "Dealing with Death Under Hospice Care." *San Mateo Times,* May 11, 1978.

Caylor, Ron. "I Beat Incurable Cancer With My Will Power." *National Enquirer,* February 13, 1979.

Chao, Stephen. "Accidental Discovery That Saved John Wayne From A Quick Death From Cancer." *National Enquirer,* July 18, 1978.

Chapin, Dwight. "The Trouper." *San Francisco Examiner & Chronicle,* September 17, 1978.

Chapman, A. H. *Put Offs and Come Ons.* New York: Putnam.

Chatfield-Taylor, Joan. "Can You Cure Yourself Of Cancer?" *San Francisco Chronicle,* March 18, 1977.

Cherry, Laurence. "On The Real Benefits of Eustress." (Interview with Dr. Hans Selye). *Psychology Today,* March 1978.

Chester, Mark. "And A Little Help From His Friends." *San Francisco Chronicle.* (California Living), March 5, 1978.

Cimons, Marlene. "Blind Photographer Finds A Way To See." *San Francisco Chronicle,* December 11, 1978.

Cimons, Marlene. "How A Dying Woman Rages Against Her Fate." *San Francisco Chronicle,* July 18, 1978.

Cleland, Max. "Breakthrough," *Guideposts,* October 1978.

Clements, David. "Car Crash Left Me Paralyzed, Speechless And Near Death—But My Will To Live Helped Me Walk and Talk Again." *National Enquirer.*

Collier, Peter. "The Old Man And The C." *New West Magazine,* April 24, 1978.

Cousins, Norman. *Anatomy of an Illness as Perceived by the Patient: Reflections on Healing and Regeneration.* New York: W. W. Norton, 1979.

Cousins, Norman. *Anatomy of an Illness as Perceived by the Patient: Reflections on Healing and Regeneration.* New York, W. W. Norton, 1979.

de Caussade, Jean-Pierre. *Abandonment To Divine Providence.* New York: Doubleday, 1975.

Eareckson, Joni. *Joni.* Grand Rapids, MI: Zondervan, 1976.

Erickson, Erik. *Childhood and Society.* New York: W. W. Norton, 1950.

Falls, Joe. "Handicapped Athletes In Wheelchairs 'Ran' 26 Mile Marathon." *National Enquirer,* February 15, 1977.

Freese, Arthur S. *Pain.* New York: Putnam, 1974.

Fry, William and Melanie Allen. *Make 'Em Laugh.* Palo Alto, CA: Science and Behavior Books, 1975.

Gifford, Frank and Charles Mangel. "Doctor Said He'd Never Walk Again, But Courage Put Paralyzed Football Player Back In The Sport." *National Enquirer,* February 8, 1977.

Goldberger, Paul. "Landmark Library Created For The Handicapped." *San Francisco Chronicle,* September 26, 1978.

Golding, George. "Coping With Terminal Illness At Home." *San Mateo Times,* June 25, 1976.

Goldsmith, Joel S. *The Art of Meditations.* New York: Harper and Row, 1956.

Goleman, Daniel. "We Are Breaking The Silence About Death." *Psychology Today,* September 1976.

Gordon, Ernest. *Through The Valley Of The Kwai.* New York: Harper and Row, 1962.

Gorney, Cynthia. "The Incredible Mayor Of Crested Butte." *San Francisco Chronicle,* April 12, 1978.

Gottlieb, Bill. "A Patient Is Not A Machine With A Broken Part." *Prevention Magazine,* June 1978.

Graedon, Joe. *The People's Pharmacy.* New York: St. Martin's Press, 1976.

Greenfield, Josh. *A Place For Noah.* New York: Holt, Rinehart and Winston, 1978.

Gurfield, Mitchell. "On Teaching Death And Dying." *Media and Methods,* February 1977.

Hamilton, Mildred. "The Family Success Story Of A Paraplegic." *San Francisco Chronicle and Examiner,* February 29, 1976.

Hamlin, Jesse. "Volunteer Handicapped Walk Away." *San Francisco Chronicle,* September 20, 1978.

Haney, Daniel. "Child With Cancer: Parents' Dilemma." *San Francisco Examiner and Chronicle,* May 7, 1978.

Hanner, Richard. "Shop For A Doctor-Like Shopping For A New Car?" *Redwood City Tribune,* November 16, 1978.

Harris, Thomas A. *I'm OK—You're OK.* New York: Harper and Row, 1967.

"He Baffled Science." *San Francisco Chronicle,* May 31, 1977.

Hines, William. "An Easier Way Of Death For Victims Of Cancer." *San Francisco Examiner and Chronicle,* August 29, 1976.

Home Nursing Textbook. American National Red Cross, 1958.

"How Placebos Work—New UC Findings." *San Francisco Chronicle,* August 29, 1978.

Howell, Mary. *Healing At Home: A Guide To Health Care For Children.* Beacon Press, 1978.

Hutschnecker, A. A. *The Will To Live.* New York: Thomas Y. Crowell, 1953.

Jacobsen, David C. *Clarity In Prayer.* Omega Books, 1976.

Jacobsen, Edmund. *You Must Relax.* New York: McGraw-Hill, 1957.

Jett, Jim. "Taking The Hard Middle Ground." *Medical Economics,* December 13, 1976.

Joffee, Linda B. "A Different Way Of Touching." *San Francisco Chronicle* (California Living), July 23, 1978.

Jordan, Lynette. "Hospice In America." *Coevolution Quarterly,* Summer 1977.

Kleinberg, David. "Waiting For The End." *San Francisco Examiner and Chronicle,* March 20, 1977.

Knoble, John. "Living.To The End." *Modern Maturity,* August-September 1977.

Kubler-Ross, Elisabeth. *Death, The Final Stage Of Growth.* Englewood Cliffs, NJ: Prentice-Hall, 1975.

Kubler-Ross, Elisabeth. "Death Does Not Exist." *Coevolution Quarterly.* Summer 1977, pages 100-107.

Kubler-Ross, Elisabeth and Mal Warshaw. *To Live Until We Say Good-Bye.* Englewood Cliffs, NJ: Prentice-Hall, 1978.

Kubler-Ross, Elisabeth. "Death Does Not Exist." *Coevolution Quarterly.* Summer 1977, pages 100-107.

Kubler-Ross, Elisabethand Mal Warshaw. *To Live Until We Say Good-Bye.* Englewood Cliffs, N.J.: Prentice-Hall, 1978.

Lamerton, Richard. *Care Of The Dying.* R. L. Sassone, 1973.

Langeley, Roger. "Americans Are Not Dumping The Aged Into Institutions." *The National Enquirer,* August 29, 1978.

Leary, Kevin. "A Blind Athlete's Victories." *San Francisco Chronicle,* October 12, 1978.

Lamerton, Richard. *Care Of The Dying.* R. L. Sassone, 1973.

Langeley, Roger. "Americans Are Not Dumping The Aged Into Institutions." *The National Enquirer,* August 29, 1978.

Leary, Kevin. "A Blind Athlete's Victories." *San Francisco Chronicle,* October 12, 1978.

Leshan, Lawrence. *You Can Fight For Your Life.* New York: M. Evans, 1977.

"Let Feisty Old Ladies Be, Expert On Nursing Advises." *Los Angeles Times,* August 17, 1978.

Linn, Amy. "New Method Reported To Help 'Lazy Eyes'." *San Francisco Chronicle,* August 23, 1978.

Malkin, Mort. "Chasing Away The Presurgery Jitters With Poetry." *Prevention,* June 1978.

McKinney, Joan. "Cancer: Her Enemy And Her Cause." *Oakland Tribune,* October 27, 1974.

Mines, Samuel. *The Conquest Of Pain.* New York: Grosset and Dunlap, 1974.

Mohr, Beth. "She Counsels Patients Who Are Dying." *San Mateo Times,* January 25, 1978.

Moody, Raymond A., Jr. *Laugh After Laugh.* Headwaters Press, 1978.

Moody, Raymond A., Jr. *Life After Life.* St. Simons Island, GA, Mockingbird Books, 1975.

Morch, Albert. "Playing A Game To Find The Right Words." *San Francisco Examiner and Chronicle,* November 19, 1978.

Moses, Kenneth L. "Effects Of The Developmental Disability On Parenting The Handicapped Child." Julia S. Molloy Education Center, 1978.

Murphy, Joseph. *The Power Of Your Subconscious Mind.* Englewood Cliffs, NJ: Prentice-Hall, 1963.

Nellis, Muriel. "Accidental Drug Addiction." *Harpers Bazaar,* August 1978.

Newsletter for Donors to St. Jude Children's Research Hospital. Volume 10, Number 2. July 1978.

Oyle, Irving. *The Healing Mind.* New York: Pocket Books, 1976.

Pauling, Linus Institute. *Newsletter,* Fall 1978.

Pelletier, K. R. *MInd As Healer, Mind As Slayer.* New York: Delta, 1977.

Pepper, Claude. "Health Care For The Elderly—At Home." *San Francisco Chronicle,* June 4, 1978.

Pettit, Charles. "Trauma Center's Fight For Life." *San Francisco Chronicle,* October 13, 1978.

Porter, Sylvia. "Home Health Care Programs." *San Francisco Chronicle,* May 17, 1978.

Porter, Sylvia. "The Movement In Home Health Care." *San Francisco Chronicle,* February 13, 1978.

Porter, Sylvia. "Jobs To Boom In Home Health Care." *San Francisco Chronicle, May 18, 1978.*

"Reconstructive Surgery." *San Francisco Chronicle,* October 15, 1978.

"Risks Posed By Mentally Sick Doctors." *San Francisco Chronicle,* January 4, 1979. From UPI.

Roberts, Oral. "I Believe The Cure For Cancer Has A Spiritual Origin." *Abundant Life,* January 1977.

Rosenbaum, Ernest H. *Living With Cancer.* New York: Praeger, 1975.

Rosenfeld, Isadore. "Choosing A Doctor You Can Trust." *San Francisco Chronicle,* July 11, 1978.

Rosenfeld, Stephen S. *The Time Of Their Dying.* New York: W. W. Norton, 1977.

Saltus, Richard. "Helping Doctors Understand The Patient As Well As The Disease." *San Francisco Chronicle,* December 24, 1978.

Scharlach, Bernice. "Back To School The Hard Way." *San Francisco Chronicle,* September 10, 1978.

Seliger, Susan. "How To Stop Killing Yourself." *San Francisco Chronicle,* September 27, 1978.

Selye, Hans. *Stress Without Distress.* New York: J. B. Lippincott, 1974.

Selye, Hans. *The Stress Of Life.* New York: McGraw-Hill. 1956.

Shealy, C. Norman, M.D. *The Pain Game.* Millbrae, CA: Celestial Arts, 1976.

Simonton, O. Carl, Stephanie Matthews Simonton, and James Creighton. *Getting Well Again.* Los Angeles: J. P. Tarcher, 1978.

Smith, Ray. "1.5 Million Americans Are Living Proof That Cancer Can Be Beaten." *National Enquirer*. June 27, 1978.

Solkoff, Joel. "What's It Like To Have Cancer?" *San Francisco Chronicle*, July 7, 1978.

Solzhenitsyn, A. *The Cancer Ward*. New York: Dial Press, 1968.

Standard First Aid And Personal Safety, The American Red Cross. New York: Doubleday, 1973.

Stark, John. "Painter Clayton Turner: Art Born Of Tragedy." *San Francisco Examiner*, March 13, 1977.

Stein, Ruth. "Laurellee Westaway: An Actress' Comeback In One Act." *San Francisco Chronicle*, September 30, 1978.

Stern, Edward L. *Prescription Drugs And Their Side Effects*. New York: Grosset and Dunlap, 1975.

Stoddard, Sandol. *The Hospice Movement*. Briarcliff Manor, NY: Stein and Day, 1978.

"Interview With Tom Ferguson." *The Mother Earth News*. Number 51, May/June 1978.

"The Trauma Of Injury In Trunkey's Ward." *San Francisco Chronicle*, October 15, 1978.

Torchia, Joseph. "One Hospital's Retreat For Parents In Need." *San Francisco Chronicle*, October 4, 1978.

Troeger, Thomas H. *Meditation: Escape To Reality*. Philadelphia: Westminster Press, 1977.

Truman, Rev. W. Lee. "Twenty Third Psalm Prescribed As Cure For Life's Ills." *The National Reporter*, September 1978.

Wallace, Marjorie and Michael Robson. *On Giant's Shoulders:* New York: Times Books, 1976.

Welles, Darla. "Housewife's Story Of A Victory." *San Jose Mercury*. February 1, 1976.

White, Jane See. "A Merciful Death Watch Inside The Home." *San Mateo Times*, August 12, 1978. From AP.

Will, George F. "A Good Death." *Newsweek*, January 9, 1978.

Woodward, Kenneth (and staff). "Living With Dying." *Newsweek*, May 1, 1978.

Wright, H. T. *The Matthew Tree*. New York: Pantheon Books, 1975.

Yarish, Alice. "A Family Celebration Of A Victory Over Leukemia." *San Francisco Chronicle*, September 24, 1978.

Index